Available From the American Academy of Pediatrics

Baby and Toddler Basics: Expert Answers to Parents' Top 150 Questions

The CALM Baby Method: Solutions for Fussy Days and Sleepless Nights

Caring for Your Baby and Young Child: Birth to Age 5*

Dad to Dad: Parenting Like a Pro

Guide to Toilet Training

Heading Home With Your Newborn: From Birth to Reality

High Five Discipline: Positive Parenting for Happy, Healthy, Well-Behaved Kids

My Child Is Sick! Expert Advice for Managing Common Illnesses and Injuries

The New Baby Blueprint: Caring for You and Your Little One

New Mother's Guide to Breastfeeding

Raising an Organized Child: 5 Steps to Boost Independence, Ease Frustration, and Promote Confidence

Raising Twins: Parenting Multiples From Pregnancy Through the School Years

Retro Baby: Timeless Activities to Boost Development Without All the Gear!

Sleep: What Every Parent Needs to Know

Understanding the NICU: What Parents of Preemies and Other Hospitalized Newborns Need to Know

The Working Mom Blueprint: Winning at Parenting Without Losing Yourself

Your Baby's First Year*

For additional parenting resources, visit the HealthyChildren bookstore at https://shop.aap.org/for-parents.

healthy children.org
Powered by pediatricians. Trusted by parents.
from the American Academy of Pediatrics

*This book is also available in Spanish.

UNDERSTANDING THE
NICU

What Parents of **Preemies** and Other Hospitalized Newborns Need to Know

2nd Edition

Meera Meerkov, MD, FAAP, Editor in Chief

Gary Weiner, MD, FAAP, Contributing Editor

Jeanette Zaichkin, RN, MN, NNP-BC, Contributing Editor

American Academy of Pediatrics

DEDICATED TO THE HEALTH OF ALL CHILDREN®

American Academy of Pediatrics Publishing Staff

Mary Lou White, *Chief Product and Services Officer/SVP, Membership, Marketing, and Publishing*

Mark Grimes, *Vice President, Publishing*

Holly Kaminski, *Editor, Consumer Publishing*

Caroline Heller, *PhD, Editorial Assistant*

Jason Crase, *Senior Manager, Production and Editorial Services*

Shannan Martin, *Production Manager, Consumer Publications*

Sara Hoerdeman, *Marketing and Acquisitions Manager, Consumer Products*

Published by the American Academy of Pediatrics

345 Park Blvd
Itasca, IL 60143
Telephone: 630/626-6000
Facsimile: 847/434-8000
www.aap.org

The American Academy of Pediatrics is an organization of 67,000 primary care pediatricians, pediatric medical subspecialists, and pediatric surgical specialists dedicated to the health, safety, and well-being of all infants, children, adolescents, and young adults.

The information contained in this publication should not be used as a substitute for the medical care and advice of your pediatrician. There may be variations in treatment that your pediatrician may recommend based on individual facts and circumstances.

Statements and opinions expressed are those of the authors and not necessarily those of the American Academy of Pediatrics.

Any websites, brand names, products, or manufacturers are mentioned for informational and identification purposes only and do not imply an endorsement by the American Academy of Pediatrics (AAP). The AAP is not responsible for the content of external resources. Information was current at the time of publication.

The publishers have made every effort to trace the copyright holders for borrowed materials. If they have inadvertently overlooked any, they will be pleased to make the necessary arrangements at the first opportunity.

This publication has been developed by the American Academy of Pediatrics. The contributors are expert authorities in the field of pediatrics. No commercial involvement of any kind has been solicited or accepted in the development of the content of this publication. Disclosures: All editors report no disclosures.

Every effort is made to keep *Understanding the NICU: What Parents of Preemies and Other Hospitalized Newborns Need to Know* consistent with the most recent advice and information available from the American Academy of Pediatrics.

Special discounts are available for bulk purchases of this publication. Email Special Sales at nationalaccounts@aap.org for more information.

Printed in the United States of America
9-489   1 2 3 4 5 6 7 8 9 10
CB0133
ISBN: 978-1-61002-665-9
eBook: 978-1-61002-667-3
EPUB: 978-1-61002-666-6
Cover design by Scott Rattray Design
Publication design by LSD Design, LLC
Cover photography by Gigi O'Dea, Gigi Fine Art Portraits. Reproduced with permission.
Original artwork on page 288 by Anthony Alex Letourneau. Reproduced with permission.
Library of Congress Control Number: 2023904270

Praise for the First Edition of *Understanding the NICU*

∽

"(NICU) parents need all the help they can get. Here is that support,
written in a factual yet personable voice by NICU practitioners. . . .
The stories of parents throughout will go miles in providing hope and understanding. . . .
This is an important acquisition for all collections."

—Library Journal, starred review

∽

"It's hard to imagine a better guide for parents of premature babies than this title from
the American Academy of Pediatrics."

—Booklist

∽

"A book specifically designed for parents of infants in the neonatal intensive care unit
(NICU), this book provides the essential tools that they need to navigate
their child's stay in this specialized care environment. . . . This is a high-quality book. . . .
It can serve as a navigating tool for all parents and help them to
better understand the NICU journey."

—Doody's Reviews

∽

"A valuable resource for parents and other family members as they
navigate their own NICU journey."

—Neonatal Network: The Journal of Neonatal Nursing

∽

"This is an outstanding resource for NICU parents and for their close families."

—Library Aware

"Written with parents for parents, *Understanding the NICU* provides a summary of the realities that the emotional roller coaster of NICU care will bring, the victories that babies and families enjoy, and the outcomes that NICU babies and families can anticipate. Complete and nuanced, this book will help address questions, relieve anxiety, and inform parents during their baby's NICU stay."

F. Sessions Cole, MD
Park J. White, MD, Professor of Pediatrics and Director of the Division of Newborn Medicine, Washington University School of Medicine and St. Louis Children's Hospital

"*Understanding the NICU* is a fantastic resource for NICU families. I love how it clearly explains so many NICU processes to parents who are immersed in that new environment. This book provides clear and vital information to families during a time of high stress with the birth of a premature or ill newborn. Every family will appreciate this book, both before and after delivery."

Marya Strand, MD, MS, FAAP
Associate Professor of Pediatrics, Saint Louis University School of Medicine;
Member, NRP Steering Committee

"*Understanding the NICU: What Parents of Preemies and Other Hospitalized Newborns Need to Know* is an essential go-to guide for all parents trying to navigate the complex, and sometimes overwhelming, world of the NICU. This easy-to-understand book has the perfect balance of reliable need-to-know medical information, helpful tips on navigating your baby's NICU stay, and hopeful stories of families 'who have been there.'

Unfamiliar terminology and complex NICU medical problems are simplified so parents can understand them, feel better prepared to communicate with their baby's care team, and participate in important decision-making.

Equally detailed attention is given to suggestions for successful parenting in the NICU environment.

But the standout feature of this book are the stories and pictures of real NICU babies and families interwoven with the medical information. These stories offer important encouragement and make the technical information more relatable.

A must-read for parents of NICU babies!

Linda McCarney, MSN, APRN, NNP-BC
Coordinator of NNP Education, Children's Hospital Colorado

American Academy of Pediatrics Reviewers

Susan W. Aucott, MD, FAAP

James J. Cummings, MD, FAAP

Beth Ellen Davis, MD, MPH, FAAP

Eric C. Eichenwald, MD, FAAP

Jay P. Goldsmith, MD, FAAP

Lisa Grisham, MS, NP

Charleta Guillory, MD, FAAP

Ivan Hand, MD, FAAP

Tim Jancelewicz, MD, FAAP

David Kaufman, MD, FAAP

Erin L. Keels, MS, APRN, NNP-BC

Ashley Lucke, MD, FAAP

Camilia Martin, MD, FAAP

Lawrence M. Noble, MD, FAAP

Margaret Parker, MD, FAAP

Brenda Poindexter, MD, MS, FAAP

Arun Kumar Pramanik, MD, FAAP

Karen M. Puopolo, MD, PhD, FAAP

Dan L. Stewart, MD, FAAP

Kristi Watterberg, MD, FAAP

To parents of babies who require newborn intensive care.

Find strength in knowledge. Face challenges with teamwork.

Celebrate each step forward.

Contents

. . . . . .

Family Story Icons

· · · · · · · · · · ·

This page guides you to each family's personal photos, memories, and advice about parenting in the NICU. Find these family icons throughout the book and follow their unique journey as they provide guidance and support for your experience. Also included is an update from some of the families from the first edition. You will find those in "Where Are They Now?" in the Appendix.

 Abel
22 weeks, 5 days
Family Story: pages 227–230
Chapters 1, 4, 5, 6, 7, 8, 9, 10

 Alexander (Alex)
26 weeks
Family Story: pages 153–156
Chapters 1, 3, 5

 Allison & Reece
33 weeks
Family Story: pages 291–293
Where Are They Now?: Appendix
Chapters 5, 7

 August (Auggie)
24 weeks
Family Story: pages 93–95
Where Are They Now?: Appendix
Chapters 1, 3, 5, 6, 8, 9, 10

 Bailey Jo & Abraham
32 weeks, 5 days
Family Story: pages 1–3
Chapter 8

 Christopher
32 weeks
Family Story: pages 9–11

 Colson
35 weeks
Family Story: pages 119–121
Chapters 1, 2, 3, 6, 10

 Eliana
23 weeks
Family Story: pages 35–38
Chapters 1, 2, 3, 4, 6, 7, 8, 9, 10

 Ellie
39 weeks
Family Story: pages 157–161
Chapters 2, 3, 4, 6, 8, 10

 Frankie
29 weeks
Family Story: pages 163–165
Where Are They Now?: Appendix
Chapters 1, 3, 5

 Holland & Eden
24 weeks, 3 days
Family Story: pages 123–126
Where Are They Now?: Appendix
Chapters 4, 6, 7, 8, 9, 10

Isaac & **Eliza**
27 weeks, 3 days
Family Story: pages 59–63
Chapters 1, 3, 4, 5, 6, 8, 10

 Meridith
31 weeks, 5 days
Family Story: pages 87–91
Chapters 1, 2, 6, 7, 10

 Jack (29 weeks) & **Henry** (31 weeks)
Family Story: pages 295–297
Where Are They Now?: Appendix
Chapter 5

 Nathan
24 weeks, 4 days
Family Story: pages 65–67
Chapter 8

 Kellan
32 weeks
Family Story: pages 5–7
Where Are They Now?: Appendix
Chapters 1, 2, 5, 10

 Niklas, Gabbie, & **Lukas**
28 weeks, 4 days
Family Story: pages 261–263
Where Are They Now?: Appendix
Chapter 6

 Logan
34 weeks
Family Story: pages 195–198
Chapters 1, 2, 4, 9, 10

 Pascal
41 weeks, 2 days
Family Story: pages 69–71
Where Are They Now?: Appendix
Chapters 3, 4, 6, 8, 9

 Lucy
29 weeks
Family Story: pages 39–41
Where Are They Now?: Appendix
Chapters 1, 2, 5, 6, 7, 8, 9

 Sienna
31 weeks, 4 days
Family Story: pages 231–233
Where Are They Now?: Appendix
Chapters 3, 7

 Maxwell
34 weeks
Family Story: pages 199–201

Equity, Diversity, and Inclusion Statement

The American Academy of Pediatrics is committed to principles of equity, diversity, and inclusion in its publishing program. Editorial boards, author selections, and author transitions (publication succession plans) are designed to include diverse voices that reflect society as a whole. Editor and author teams are encouraged to actively seek out diverse authors and reviewers at all stages of the editorial process. Publishing staff are committed to promoting equity, diversity, and inclusion in all aspects of publication writing, review, and production.

Please Note

We understand the importance of language and that language preferences are individual decisions. In much of this book, we have chosen to be inclusive of all people who give birth and parent babies by using gender-neutral language whenever possible. In this way, we support equitable, inclusive care to a diverse population of NICU families.

Acknowledgments

Thanks to the American Academy of Pediatrics publishing staff, who believe in this book and its potential to help NICU parents navigate their journey.

Thank you to the many people who contributed to the photographs for this book.

Gigi O'Dea of Gigi Fine Art Portraits for contributing several amazing photographs of NICU babies and their families, including the cover photo.

Tamera Miller, RNC, NNP

A special thank you to all of the parents who contributed stories and photos of their NICU experience and beyond. Your pictures are worth a thousand words.

Thank you to the health care professionals, whose unique contributions are much appreciated.

Introduction

· · · · · · · · ·

The birth of a baby is one of the most personal, exhausting, beautiful, and emotionally charged events of a lifetime. But when everything does not go as expected—if labor is complicated or your baby is born preterm or facing serious complications—different emotions take over. If your baby is now in the neonatal intensive care unit (NICU), you may be feeling anxious, confused, guilty, angry, and even sad over the loss of the uncomplicated, healthy birth experience you had envisioned.

This book can help you understand the NICU and how you can best meet this challenge. It was written by professionals with decades of NICU experience in partnership with 23 families whose babies spent their first weeks, and sometimes months, in the NICU. Each family's story is unique, yet they all share common themes of strength and determination. Every parent was afraid, but they all learned to navigate the complex world of the NICU and become valuable members of their baby's health care team. You will learn, through their words, about the NICU parent experience—from birth, through intensive care, to homecoming, and beyond.

We invite you to become an important member of your baby's health care team. We believe parents can and should play an active role in their baby's care. This book was written for parents who want to learn about their baby's illness, how to overcome the barriers to parenting in the NICU, and how to nurture their NICU graduate at home.

You will not need all the information in this book because your baby will not have every problem described here. Look at the table of contents to find the sections that interest you most— and know that what interests you will change as your baby progresses through hospitalization. As you read through the sections that pertain to your baby, you may notice some parts of your baby's treatment are somewhat different than what is described here. That is because treatment approaches vary across the country and nursing and medical research is constantly changing the way babies in the NICU are managed. Ask your baby's team about any differences that concern you.

As you read the stories of families who volunteered to share their experiences, you will notice that some families have recent NICU experience, while others have NICU graduates who are already in school. All of these parents agreed to share their intensely personal stories so they could give you hope on your journey and help you discover your own strengths during hospitalization and as your child grows. A complete list of all the family stories is included on page xiii.

The NICU can be a place of remarkable healing. You will meet other parents whose support will give you strength. You will meet health care professionals who have devoted their careers to helping babies like yours. You will discover that the NICU offers a unique blend of technology and compassion that encourages healing and growth not only for babies, but also for parents. Learning to be a good parent never ends. We hope you get a good start here.

Meera Meerkov, MD, FAAP
Gary Weiner, MD, FAAP
Jeanette Zaichkin, RN, MN, NNP-BC

Bailey Jo
&
Abraham

Born at 32 weeks, 5 days

Mom cuddles Abraham and Bailey Jo.

Dad enjoys some skin-to-skin time.

Bailey Jo and Abraham were born at 32 weeks 5 days of gestation due to preeclampsia. I remember the first time I saw them—I had to wait until I was out of recovery from my cesarean. They were so tiny. Abraham weighed 4 pounds 1 ounce and Bailey Jo weighed 3 pounds 10 ounces. I wasn't allowed to hold them; I could stick my hand into the incubator and touch them. I remember crying and feeling so helpless.

Abraham was treated for mild respiratory distress and required nasal high-flow oxygen. Bailey Jo's respiratory distress was a little more of a concern and she was on a continuous positive airway pressure (CPAP) machine for the first 8 days until she was weaned to room air. Both were treated with phototherapy for jaundice. Both babies were also treated for apnea of prematurity, which was very scary. They would just stop breathing and an alarm would go off and nurses would run in, jiggle the babies a little, and then they would breathe again. That became normal for us, and it got to the point where the alarm would go off and by the time the nurses arrived, we had gotten them breathing. The twins also needed feeding support and had nasogastric (NG) tubes.

The first time I held them was so scary. They had all these tubes and cords and monitors hooked up to them. The nurses were so kind and not only caring for our tiny babies, but for me as well. We live 60 miles away from the hospital; I stayed in special housing, which allowed me to be with the babies every day. My husband worked during the week and would come down every weekend, bringing our oldest, Lydia, who was 7 at the time. I would get up every morning and get to the hospital before rounds and leave after the shift change between 8:00 and 8:30 pm. I didn't want to miss anything. I remember one of the nurses telling me I had to eat and take a nap. She even went to the cafeteria and got me lunch. The nurses became like family. They listened, they loved our babies, and they were our biggest advocates.

Abraham was released after 24 days—completely off oxygen and taking 100% of his feeds by mouth. So we had one twin released and one still in the NICU. The NICU staff were so accommodating, letting me bring Abraham to the NICU with me every day to see Bailey Jo. It was hard being away from home and family. Finally, on day 34, we had our whole family home.

Bailey Jo and Abraham at 15 months of age with their parents and big sister, Lydia.

They love music and dancing, they adore their big sister, and she loves them just as much. They are growing and changing and learning every day. We have stayed in contact with several of our nurses and stop in for visits. I have never met a more caring and compassionate group of nurses and doctors. We could not have asked for a better experience in the NICU.

Bridget and Matthew, parents of Bailey Jo and Abraham

Kellan

Born at 32 weeks

Only hours after celebrating our little miracle at his baby shower, my water broke and contractions began. Kellan Patrick joined the world at 4 pounds 13 ounces, exactly 32 weeks' gestation.

The reality of what was happening did not kick in when the contractions did. It didn't even kick in when I delivered in the operating room and my son was whisked off. It was all so

surreal and I was only thinking about the fact that I had gotten to meet the baby that I had waited for, for so long. What I had envisioned for those moments after birth was not at all what I experienced and it was hard to accept. I had to accept that other people were going to be responsible for helping my baby survive. The statement, "It will get worse before it gets better," became all too real, all too quickly.

Kellan, at 32 weeks' gestation, resting on his tummy. CPAP is attached to his face with a special headgear, while an arm board keeps his IV in place at his side.

On his second day of life, Kellan was having trouble breathing on his own, so he was intubated. It was at that exact moment that I realized how serious this whole situation was. That moment defined me as a new mom of a preemie.

This photo was taken on Kellan's first birthday. I wanted to capture another side of the journey we had been on—the side that represented him home and growing. I want to always remember, and have him know, just how special he is and how far he has come.

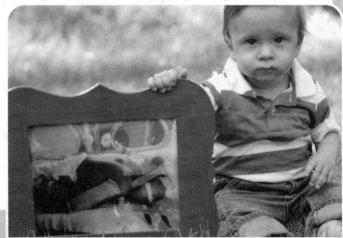

Kellan at age 1, with his NICU photo.

The following day, I was released from the hospital and had to cope with going home without my baby. In the days to follow, I was at his side from 9:00 am to 9:00 pm, participating in changing, feeding (even breastfeeding), kangarooing him, and being there to listen and learn during rounds. I was determined to take it all in and be as involved in his care and recovery as I could.

We did experience some delay in gross motor skills in the first 6 months, as well as speech delays at age 2, but we remained committed to making sure Kellan had the resources he needed to reach his milestones at his own pace. Although not accepted at 6 months of age, he was accepted into the Early On Program offered in our county and he received monthly visits from a speech therapist for 1 year.

Kellan, at age 3.

Today, Kellan is all boy and loves all things sports. He can tell you the name of all 32 NFL teams just by the look of their helmet and asks to hit balls at the golf range at every opportunity. The only thing bigger than his imagination is his heart, and he melts ours with his fun personality and his love for his little sister.

We had 37 days of ups and downs but a lifetime ahead of being grateful for the knowledge of the people around us. The dedication they had to helping Kellan survive! Our story could have been worse, and many are. We will never forget those who saved Kellan's life. They are the same people who taught us so much about the NICU journey as well as our journey as new parents. **Read more about Kellan in "Where Are They Now?" in the Appendix.**

Marnie, mother of Kellan

Christopher

Born at 32 weeks

· · · · · · · · · · · · · · ·

My son, Christopher, was born 2 months premature. At birth, Christopher weighed in at 3 pounds 14 ounces and spent 28 days in the NICU.

I had lost a baby at 5 months' gestation and then had a miscarriage in the first trimester before Christopher was born. So when Christopher was born 8 weeks premature, I was scared and thought he was going to be taken from me too. I can remember when my husband and I went to see him one night and when we arrived, we were told that the doctor wanted to see us. Her first words were, "We've been trying to call you all day," and I lost it at that point. She asked me not to get upset and only wanted to tell us that Christopher's nurse had noticed that he was sleepier than normal, so they ran a bunch of tests and discovered he had an infection that is pretty common in preemies. So Christopher was on antibiotics for the next 10 days. We were constantly on an emotional roller coaster.

He came home on oxygen and an apnea monitor for another 2 months at home. He had follow-up appointments for the apnea and soon was taken off of the monitor and oxygen.

Christopher is doing excellent in school academically. This is his fourth year in band. He plays the clarinet. Outside of the band, he is also in a jazz band taught by his band teacher. This is his third year doing that.

Christopher, at age 10 days.

When you have a child born too soon, you don't know what the outcome is going to be. You wonder if they are going to be like other children who were born healthy. Your life is different and I truly think it makes you a better person. If you weren't a strong person, you become one. That little person is depending on you.

Christine, mother of Christopher

Christopher, at age 13.

CHAPTER 1

An Unexpected Beginning

> " My original birthing plan
> included listening to soothing music,
> using my Lamaze positions to ease my
> baby through the birth canal, and using
> no pain medication—a beautiful affair that
> would gently bring Logan into our world.
> Thus far, the birth was not going
> according to plan, but in the moment,
> there was nothing I would not do to
> keep Logan safe. No fear, just action.
>
> *Christina, mother of **Logan***

Giving birth is an adventure unlike any other life experience. Most parents anticipate the big event with a mixture of excitement and apprehension, yet few are truly prepared for any complications that may result in a baby needing intensive care.

Most of the time, the circumstances that result in a high-risk birth are beyond anyone's control. Even with the best prenatal care, a neonatal intensive care unit (NICU) admission is sometimes unavoidable. No one chooses a complicated pregnancy, an early delivery, or for their newborn to be admitted to the NICU. Finding out that pregnancy, labor, and birthing may pose risks to your health or your partner's health or that your unborn baby may have health problems can be frightening. Understanding the basics of birthing "at risk" may help you cope with the stress that accompanies a different beginning.

Health Problems in Pregnancy That May Affect Your Baby

Babies develop within the complex environment of the womb *(uterus)*. This is called the baby's *prenatal environment*. The growing fetus depends on the placenta, a structure that develops between the pregnant person's uterus and baby, which provides oxygen and nutrition until birth. The placenta is attached to the fetus by the umbilical cord. This dependence means a pregnant person's health and well-being are very important to their growing baby. Alcohol, drugs (including misuse of prescription drugs), and cigarettes create a risky environment for a growing fetus. In addition, some medical conditions and pregnancy complications can affect a developing fetus. Some of the commonly monitored conditions during pregnancy include

- ▸ Diabetes
- ▸ High blood pressure
- ▸ Infection
- ▸ Blood type incompatibilities

Diabetes and How It Might Affect Your Baby

When you eat, your pancreas secretes a hormone called *insulin* that keeps your blood sugar *(blood glucose)* levels within a healthy range. Diabetes develops when the body does not make enough insulin or does not use insulin properly. When this happens, blood glucose levels can be too high.

Some people already have diabetes before they become pregnant. Others are unable to produce enough insulin, or their insulin does not work properly to control blood sugar levels when they become pregnant. This is a condition called *gestational diabetes*. In either case, the pregnant person's blood glucose may rise to higher-than-normal levels. Extra glucose easily crosses into the developing fetus and the fetal pancreas responds by producing extra insulin. Increased glucose and insulin levels change the fetal environment and can harm the developing baby. If diabetes is present before conception, the baby's organs may not develop normally and there is an increased risk of serious birth defects *(congenital anomalies)*. Higher-than-normal glucose and insulin levels later in pregnancy may cause the baby to have excess fat, breathing problems after birth, problems with low blood sugar after birth *(hypoglycemia)*, and higher risks of obesity and diabetes later in life. If you have diabetes, your baby's health depends on keeping your blood glucose level within a healthy range before conception and throughout your pregnancy.

High Blood Pressure and How It Might Affect Your Baby

Blood pressure usually does not increase during pregnancy, but high blood pressure (*hypertension*) does complicate about 6% to 17% of pregnancies in the United States and can cause health problems for both the pregnant person and the developing fetus.

- If you had high blood pressure before becoming pregnant or develop high blood pressure before 20 weeks of gestation, it is called *chronic hypertension.*
- If you had normal blood pressure before pregnancy but develop high blood pressure for the first time after 20 weeks of gestation, it is called *gestational hypertension.*

Hypertension during pregnancy increases the risk of preterm birth, cesarean birth, premature separation of the placenta from the uterus (*placental abruption)*, and a complication called *preeclampsia.*

Preeclampsia occurs when, in addition to high blood pressure, there are signs that other organs are not working normally. In addition to hypertension, a common sign of preeclampsia is protein leaking from the kidneys into the urine. Preeclampsia may progress to more severe conditions, including *HELLP syndrome* and *eclampsia.* HELLP stands for *h*emolysis (breakdown of red blood cells [RBCs]), *e*levated *l*iver enzymes, and *l*ow *p*latelets. If someone with preeclampsia develops seizures, the condition is called *eclampsia.* HELLP syndrome and eclampsia can be life-threatening conditions for the pregnant person and fetus.

If gestational hypertension develops, medications may be prescribed to lower blood pressure. The doctor may recommend additional testing and will monitor the baby's growth for the remainder of the pregnancy. If blood pressure stays high, blood flow to the pregnant person's kidneys, liver, brain, and uterus can be reduced. This can limit the baby's supply of oxygen and nutrients and reduce fetal growth. The doctor may recommend early delivery if severe high blood pressure develops that does not respond to treatment, if there are signs of severe preeclampsia, or if the baby is showing signs of poor growth.

Infection During Pregnancy and How It Might Affect Your Baby

Infections during pregnancy that affect the developing fetus are most commonly caused by bacteria, viruses, or, very rarely, a fungus or a parasite. Although many infections that occur during pregnancy will resolve without causing any harm to the developing baby, some organisms can cross the placenta and cause a congenital infection that harms developing organs. Among the risks are preterm birth, miscarriage, abnormal fetal growth and development, abnormal fetal blood cell counts, jaundice, seizures, and pneumonia. Many of these infections can be prevented by being up to date on immunizations before pregnancy and following good health practices to decrease exposure to infections. Even with good health care, some infections during pregnancy cannot be prevented and may affect the baby. Common newborn infections are discussed in Chapter 4.

COVID-19 Infection During Pregnancy

Since the declaration of the COVID-19 pandemic in March 2020, there has been concern regarding how this novel virus affects pregnant people and their babies. The most up-to-date data show that pregnant people infected with COVID-19 are at risk for developing more severe symptoms and are at increased risk for pregnancy complications that can affect their babies' health such as preterm birth. However, it is uncommon for the baby to be affected with COVID-19 during the pregnancy, and infants born to people with COVID-19 infections do not typically have any immediate health problems directly attributable to the virus. The possibility that babies exposed

to COVID-19 during pregnancy may have a higher risk of developmental problems is still being investigated. Although the current data are reassuring, we believe it is important for pregnant people to protect themselves from getting infected with COVID-19. Receiving the COVID-19 vaccine before, during, or after pregnancy has been shown to decrease the risk of developing the disease and reduces the severity of the disease in breakthrough cases. When given to a pregnant person, the vaccine has no known risks for the fetus or baby. We are continuing to learn more about COVID-19 infections during and shortly after pregnancy. If you had a COVID-19 infection and are concerned about possible effects on your baby, speak with your pediatrician.

Please use this QR code to go directly to www.cdc.gov/coronavirus/ 2019-ncov/vaccines/ recommendations/ pregnancy.html.

Blood Type Incompatibility and How It Might Affect Your Baby

All humans have substances attached to the surface of their RBCs called blood group *antigens*. The specific combination of antigens determines your blood type, which is described by a series of letters and names, such as blood type A-positive. The most commonly discussed parts of your blood type are the ABO system and the Rh (positive or negative) system. Blood group antigens, and your blood type, are inherited, with a portion coming from each of your parents. If parents have more than 1 child, each child may inherit a unique combination of antigens and have a different blood type.

Your immune system protects your body from "foreign" cells by creating antibodies. If a baby's RBCs have an antigen that the pregnant person's blood does not, the pregnant person's immune system may identify the baby's blood as "foreign" and produce antibodies that cross the placenta and destroy fetal blood cells. These are called incompatible blood types.

Most commonly, this happens if the pregnant person is type O and the baby is type A or type B (*ABO incompatible*) or if the pregnant person is Rh-negative and the baby is Rh-positive (*Rh incompatible*). Rh incompatibility usually does not affect an Rh-negative person's first pregnancy because their immune system has not been activated yet. ABO incompatibility may affect the first pregnancy for a type O person because they often already have anti-A and anti-B antibodies even without exposure to fetal blood during pregnancy. In addition to the ABO and Rh groups, RBCs have other "minor" antigens that may cause incompatibility.

Blood group incompatibilities can cause the fetus to have a low RBCs count (become *anemic*). Usually, ABO incompatibility causes milder disease than Rh incompatibility. Severe fetal anemia before birth occurs in only about 1% of all ABO-incompatible pregnancies. But if the pregnant person's antibody response against their fetus is very strong, as is often the case with Rh incompatibility, RBC destruction may cause severe anemia before birth. High-risk pregnancies with known blood group incompatibilities are monitored via ultrasound for signs of severe anemia. Sometimes, the fetus will develop swelling and signs of heart failure (*fetal hydrops*) and will need to receive blood transfusions before birth.

Because Rh incompatibility is preventable and causes serious complications for the fetus and newborn, pregnant people who are Rh-negative are followed very closely throughout their pregnancies. An injected medication called Rho(D) immune globulin *(RhoGAM [WinRho* in Canada]) is given at the beginning of the third trimester and after any procedure that causes fetal blood to cross into the pregnant person's bloodstream. RhoGAM may block the pregnant person's immune system from producing antibodies against fetal RBCs, but it is effective only if antibodies have not already formed.

Fetal Factors That Affect Your Baby

Gestational Age

Gestational age is the number of weeks that have elapsed between the first day of the pregnant person's last menstrual period and the current date. By asking, "What is the baby's gestational

age?" the health care provider can determine if the baby is term, preterm, or post-term. Gestational age is correlated with birth weight, length, and measurement of the head to categorize the baby's size as appropriate for gestational age *(AGA)*, small for gestational age *(SGA)*, or large for gestational age *(LGA)*.

Eliana, 10 days old in this photo, is an extremely preterm newborn. Eliana's father will cover her with a warm blanket to continue skin-to-skin care.

What Is Gestational Age?

Gestational age determines whether a newborn is term (on time), preterm (born early), or post-term (born late). A baby born before 37 weeks' gestation is preterm; however, gestational ages can be described in the following periods:

- **Extremely preterm:** born before 28 weeks of pregnancy
- **Very preterm:** born between 28 and 32 weeks of pregnancy
- **Moderately preterm:** born between 32 and 34 weeks of pregnancy
- **Late preterm:** born between 34 and 36 weeks of pregnancy
- **Early term:** born between 37 and 39 weeks of pregnancy
- **Full term:** born between 39 and 41 weeks of pregnancy
- **Late term:** born between 41 and 42 weeks of pregnancy
- **Post-term (also called postdates):** born after 42 weeks of pregnancy

Gestational age is usually determined by the date of the last menstrual period. However, this date may be uncertain. Ultrasound in the first trimester of pregnancy is accurate in predicting the due date within 3 to 5 days. After that, ultrasound estimates a due date within 1 or 2 weeks.

Multiple-Gestation Pregnancies

If there is more than 1 baby (called a *multiple-gestation pregnancy*), lack of space in the uterus can affect 1 or more baby's weight gain during the third trimester. Through week 29 of a healthy pregnancy, the growth rates for multiple fetuses are nearly the same as those for a single fetus. But at 30 weeks of gestation and later, multiple fetuses do not gain weight as rapidly as a single fetus does.

The terms used to describe multiple-gestation pregnancies can be confusing. You may hear the terms *fraternal* and *identical* multiples. Multiples that form from a single sperm and egg are identical, while multiples that form from 2 or more different sperm and eggs are fraternal. Fraternal twins may be different genders and have very different appearance. Health professionals frequently describe multiples by the characteristics of their placenta. The part of the placenta that attaches to the uterus is called the chorion. The part of the placenta that forms the sac and holds fluid is called the amnion. Multiples may share some or all parts of the placenta, or each may have their own independent placenta. Health professionals often describe whether the fetuses share parts of the same placenta. If your babies came from a single egg, the fetuses are called *identical* and usually, but not always, share the same chorion (*monochorionic*). Most often, identical twins still have their own amniotic sac (*diamniotic*). This combination is often called "*mo-di*" twins. If your babies came from more than 1 egg, the fetuses are *not* identical and each will have their own independent placenta (*dichorionic* and *diamniotic*, called "*di-di*").

Abnormal blood flow through the placenta is a risk for identical twins who share the same chorion (*monochorionic*). This is called a *twin-to-twin transfusion.* One twin receives too much blood, while the other receives too little. The twin who gets less blood flow (the donor twin) can show signs of poor growth, anemia, poor kidney function, decreased amniotic fluid, and heart failure. The twin who receives too much blood (the recipient) is often sicker, has too much amniotic fluid, and can show signs of heart failure. Multiple-gestation pregnancies are often evaluated by ultrasound early in the pregnancy to determine if the fetuses share a portion of the placenta.

People with multiple-gestation pregnancies are also at higher risk of developing gestational diabetes, gestational hypertension, preeclampsia, and preterm birth.

> Overnight, our perfectly healthy pregnancy changed to a high-risk pregnancy with the possibility of losing both babies. It was the hardest 2 weeks and 3 days of my life because I had no idea what the outcome would be. I kept my pregnancy going until I was 27 weeks and 3 days when I had to have an emergency C-section. Isaac weighed 2 pounds 0.8 ounce, and Eliza was a little bigger, weighing in at 2 pounds 3 ounces.
>
> *Parina, mother of **Isaac** and **Eliza***

Congenital Anomalies (Birth Defects)

Because ultrasound during pregnancy is so common, physical abnormalities in a baby may be detected before birth.

The medical term for these variations is *congenital* (meaning "existing at birth") *anomalies,* and they may also be called *birth defects.* Congenital anomalies may appear as a single finding, or there may be several together. While many congenital anomalies discovered by prenatal ultrasound are minor and not expected to cause any significant problem, some congenital anomalies are significant and may cause serious or even life-threatening problems after birth. Some will have unknown significance and an uncertain effect on the baby until after the birth. It is important to note that not all congenital anomalies can be detected by ultrasound.

When a congenital anomaly is discovered before the baby's birth, parents and their health care team usually have time to discuss the findings, meet with additional experts, obtain additional tests, and prepare in advance for any special needs.

When a significant congenital anomaly is found in a baby before birth, parents are often referred to a specialized team of experts working together in a prenatal diagnosis center or clinic. Depending on the type of anomaly found, the team may include maternal-fetal medicine specialists, neonatologists, genetics experts, surgeons, pediatric subspecialists like cardiologists or nephrologists, developmental pediatricians, or palliative care pediatricians. If a congenital anomaly is found, you will learn much more about what this means and what can be done about it from this team. They will often show you pictures, videos, or models to help you understand what is happening to your baby. They may also help you connect with other parents whose babies had similar problems. Treatments for many congenital anomalies or diseases are still being developed, so you may discover that not all NICUs or specialist teams will manage a problem the same way.

Many parents want more information and will look on the internet and social media for additional details, advice, and stories from other parents. However, research has consistently shown that internet resources contain plenty of inaccurate medical information, and social media sites can also have misleading or biased medical information. Ask your medical team for recommended sources of reliable information.

> **We found out around 16 weeks of gestation that Colson had an abdominal wall abnormality. The information and references we received from the doctors helped us decide that we would continue to manage my pregnancy within our local health care system because it was closer to home, but deliver Colson at a hospital farther away that was connected to the children's hospital where he would receive intensive care.**
>
> *Jewel, mother of* **Colson**

Where Will You Give Birth?

Your baby's health may depend on decisions made before birth. By working with your team of doctors, nurses, nurse practitioners, midwives, and other health care professionals in making these decisions, you are acting as a responsible parent even before your baby is born. Your team's first recommendation may concern the hospital where your baby will be born.

Levels of Care

Your hospital's designated level of obstetric and neonatal care may affect where your baby is born. Although every hospital is equipped to handle emergencies, many smaller community hospitals prefer to transport patients with high-risk obstetric or neonatal problems to a larger medical center where staff are more experienced at managing complicated pregnancies and the care of sick newborns.

The American Academy of Pediatrics has proposed standard definitions for neonatal levels of care (levels I through IV). Interpretation and application of these levels vary across the United States, but a higher level of care means there are more intensive care specialists and services available for your newborn. If your care team determines that problems related to labor or your baby's birth may become complicated, they may recommend transfer to a hospital that offers a higher level of care before your baby is born.

> ❝ The whole experience was surreal and overwhelming. We simply didn't know what to expect from a baby born 2½ months early, and we weren't prepped, mentally or logistically, for her arrival. ❞
>
> *Matt, father of **Lucy***

When Your Baby Needs Surgery

When you first hear the words, "Your baby might need surgery," you may be overwhelmed with questions. For most parents, the most common questions are, "Will my baby be all right?"; "Who will be involved?"; "What will the surgery involve?"; and "What can I do to help?"

Not all hospitals have the experts to perform neonatal surgery. If your baby needs a special type of surgery, such as heart surgery, you may be referred to a large university medical center or a children's hospital. Transfer to another hospital, especially if it is far from your home, may present more challenges, such as transportation, more time off from work, and child care for your other children. A social worker or care coordinator at the hospital can help you navigate the system and decrease some of your stress.

Transferring to Another Hospital Before Birth: What Can You Expect?

If the pregnant parent or baby is expected to require specialized care and is at a hospital that does not offer these services, transferring to another hospital before birth may be a good idea. However, if the pregnant parent is so ill that transport would further endanger their health or if labor has progressed to the point where birth could happen during transport, transferring before birth may not be possible. In these cases, it is safer to give birth at the local hospital, stabilize the baby after birth, and then transport the baby to a specialized hospital.

Even though transferring to another hospital before birth may be necessary to obtain the care needed, it will change some of your plans. When you change hospitals, you may not have your own doctor or midwife to deliver your baby and your regular pediatrician may not be directly involved in your baby's care. You may be far from home, without the support of family and friends. If the specialized hospital is far away, it may mean making long-term arrangements to care for your household and other children. Your family may worry about your health and the uncertain health of your baby. Transport can feel like an emergency, and the nonpregnant parent may feel all the responsibility for holding things together.

During this stressful time, partners need to communicate honestly with each other, support each other, and be together, if possible, when information is provided. Stress can make it difficult to understand everything you're told. If you and your partner hear the information together, you may be better able to clarify the facts for one another.

The staff at the community hospital or a member of the transport team should provide you with directions to the medical center and its perinatal unit. Your case manager or the hospital social worker should be able to tell you about affordable lodging, parking discounts at or near the medical center, and other important information to help you navigate an unfamiliar place.

Your Care Providers

The people who attend your baby's birth will depend on the specific circumstances. When labor becomes complicated or the baby is expected to require assistance, many interventions become necessary and people with equipment rapidly fill the room.

The following list describes the care providers you may encounter during labor. Chapter 2 is devoted to helping you understand the roles of people in the NICU.

Labor Nurses

Your labor nurses are important sources of information, serve as your advocates, and provide links to the other people involved in the process of labor and birth.

Physicians

Several physicians may be involved, including obstetricians (specialists in pregnancy, labor, and delivery), perinatologists/maternal-fetal medicine doctors (specialists in high-risk obstetric and fetal medical care), anesthesiologists (specialists in pain management), and neonatologists (specialists in newborn intensive care). In a teaching hospital, medical students and physicians in training (including interns, residents, and fellows) may also be involved.

Other Hospital Personnel

In addition to your labor nurses and physicians, you may meet other specialized hospital staff. Laboratory personnel may draw blood samples; a sonographer may perform an ultrasound; and a social worker may meet with you to discuss available resources and your personal and family needs. Each member of the team provides an important aspect of hospital care.

Questions to Ask About the Plan of Care

You may have many questions about the plan of care, but because of the stressful situation, you may have difficulty remembering all of your questions. It may help to keep a journal or a note on your phone to write down all of your questions as they come to mind. Keep it with you at all times. Some questions you may have for your team include:

- How long is this hospital stay? Is hospital discharge possible before the baby is born?
- What activities are permitted? Using the restroom and shower? Or does "bed rest" mean staying in bed all the time?
- Is a regular diet served during this hospitalization or is there a special diet?
- What signs and symptoms should be reported to the nurse or doctor?
- Why might an emergency birth be necessary?
- If an emergency birth is necessary, what will happen? Who can attend the birth as the support person?

When you are nervous, it is normal to forget what you are told and not hear all of the information you are given. Write down the answers to your questions in your journal or phone so you can refer to them later. If you have more questions or have forgotten the answers, you may always ask questions again. The health care team wants you to be as comfortable as possible in this stressful situation.

What to Expect From the Health Care Team

In general, you should always expect courteous and respectful treatment. All members of your health care team should introduce themselves by name and job title before performing examinations or asking questions. Even in an emergency, team members should protect your privacy by closing hallway doors and using privacy screens. Communication may not be easy for you at this difficult time, but keep in mind that you are an important part of the team and your input is valuable.

Obstetric Care Plans

Talking with the obstetric team and asking questions will give you vital information about the care plan. Discussing this information with your partner or others you trust will help you and your health care team make the best decisions for your baby and your family.

Finding a New Plan

If you have reached the point in your pregnancy when you have planned your labor and birth experience but then find you are at risk, you may still be able to keep part of your plan. If your physician recommends a cesarean birth, for example, ask if you may play the music you planned for labor in the operating room. Having some control over your care may reduce the intensity of your feelings of loss for the "perfect" birth.

Corticosteroids

If there is a strong chance your baby will be born very preterm, your doctor may recommend treatment with *corticosteroids* (often referred to simply as *steroids*). Common choices include *betamethasone* and *dexamethasone*. Corticosteroids given to the pregnant person before birth have several important benefits for preterm newborns, including decreasing the severity of breathing problems, improving blood pressure, and decreasing the chance of bleeding in the brain. Corticosteroids work best about 48 hours after the first dose and continue to work for about 7 days. This single course of steroid therapy given to the pregnant person is safe and does not hurt the baby's growth or development.

> ❝ My team of doctors did everything they could to try and stop the labor from progressing. Within hours, they determined that our little man was coming whether we were ready or not. Our doctor came in and started going over what we could expect ... what they were hoping for but also what they were hoping would not happen. ❞

*Marnie, mother of **Kellan***

Vaginal or Cesarean Birth?

When spontaneous vaginal birth is safe, this is usually the option of choice. Vaginal birth eliminates the risks of surgical complications and shortens the postpartum hospital stay and recovery period.

Alexander, born by C-section at 26 weeks, spends a few moments with his mother Stacy before NICU admission. He has a CPAP mask in place to make breathing easier.

Any condition that causes concern about the baby's well-being, such as trouble with the fetal heart rate or serious bleeding or illness, may make cesarean birth the best choice for a healthy outcome. Other common reasons for cesarean birth include previous cesarean births, failure to make progress in labor, and unusual fetal presentation (for example, the baby is not positioned to deliver headfirst). Your health care providers' experience and training in this type of medical and nursing care will guide their clinical judgment. The information they give you is based on careful consideration of the risks and benefits of each birthing method.

If preterm labor cannot be stopped and a vaginal birth is expected, you may discover that labor and birth progress quickly. Even though vaginal birth is a natural process, an unusually fast birth (a *precipitous birth*) can be frightening. Because health care providers and equipment must move quickly, a precipitous birth often feels like an emergency. Your doctor and labor nurse will support you through the urgency of the birth. Afterward, ask them to help you review what happened and clarify details that are important to you.

A Difficult Question: "Will My Baby Live?"

"Will my baby live?" is a common question asked by parents who face a high-risk birth. This is a difficult question, and the answer depends on many factors.

If there's time before the birth, your obstetric provider and the neonatologist or pediatrician will speak with you about what to expect when your baby is born. As your baby's parent, you are expected to help make health care decisions in your baby's best interests. In most situations, you will be asked to participate in the choices and decisions that affect your baby's care at birth. If birth is about to happen or has become an emergency, it may be difficult to get all of the information you need and have time to think about your choices. This makes clear and ongoing communication with the neonatal team most important, so you can be updated on your baby's condition.

If your baby is expected to be extremely preterm, generally between 22 and 24 weeks of gestation, or if your baby is known to have a serious congenital anomaly (*birth defect*), your health care team may talk with you and your partner about your baby's chances for survival and significant complications. This helps you share in the decision-making about what kind of medical care your baby will receive during the first minutes after birth. You may have the opportunity to discuss what, if any, limits you want to consider concerning interventions for your baby after birth. Every situation is unique and, sometimes, life-prolonging measures might cause suffering without resulting in any meaningful hope for recovery. In these cases, many parents simply want to hold and comfort their baby soon after birth. You may prefer something in between, such as beginning resuscitation by providing breathing assistance and then, depending on the baby's response and the advice of the health care provider, deciding to go ahead with more complex steps or stop and provide comfort only. It is important to know that interventions can be stopped after they are started, but it is not acceptable to provide comfort only and then change the plan and start resuscitative interventions many minutes after the baby is born. A baby who survives a delayed resuscitation is at risk of serious disability.

Your NICU team cannot make any promises about what will happen after the delivery. If the baby's condition at birth is different from that expected, the plan may change. In this case, the NICU team will keep you informed about your baby's condition and may offer some choices about next steps. Sometimes, resuscitating and admitting the baby to the NICU gives you and the medical team more time to gather information about the best plan of action and gives you more time to ask important questions.

> " I was only 24 weeks' pregnant. There was nothing I could say or do to change what was about to happen. My body had failed my child. Only later would I understand this feeling of guilt more fully. There was so much more we were about to learn, about our son, about ourselves, about the exhausting and complicated journey of a baby born much too soon, about love that is deferred. "
>
> *Robyn, mother of **Auggie***

What Can Happen at Birth

Occasionally, a baby is born sick without warning. Most of the time, the obstetric and neonatal team of doctors, nurses, and respiratory therapists anticipate problems and are ready to deal with them. At every birth, members of the neonatal team work together to assess the baby's condition.

Every hospital and birthing center delivery area is equipped to provide lifesaving interventions (*resuscitation or stabilization*) to newborns. These interventions may take place in the delivery room or in a room nearby. In any case, preparing for the birth of a sick or preterm newborn brings tension into the room. A physician, a nurse practitioner, or a physician assistant usually leads the neonatal resuscitation team, and you may hear the team leader assigning duties and checking equipment. Caregivers are ready to help the newborn breathe and achieve or maintain the pulse and blood pressure necessary for life.

In many settings, the newborn receives lifesaving care in the delivery room. In other settings, a nearby room is used for evaluation and resuscitation, as pictured here.

> ❝ We knew it would be an emergency C-section. The labor and delivery staff prepared me with everything I needed to know. Afterwards, they wheeled me into the NICU on a stretcher. The nurses and doctors were connecting Frankie to all her monitors. I honestly believe I was in complete shock. I didn't hear a word they were saying. ❞

*Lisa, mother of **Frankie***

Resuscitation and Stabilization Activities

The steps taken to resuscitate a newborn depend on the baby's condition at birth and special needs.

First Steps

Immediately after birth, the obstetric care provider may cover your baby with a warm towel and suction fluids out of your baby's mouth and nose. Depending on the circumstances surrounding the birth, the obstetric provider may wait to clamp and cut the baby's umbilical cord. If the placenta is working as it should, even a short delay allows a significant amount of additional blood to flow into the newborn after birth.

After the umbilical cord is clamped and cut, the baby may be moved to the radiant warmer, which is a portable cart with a mattress and a heat source overhead. Most babies are quickly wiped dry to prevent chilling; however, preterm babies less than 32 weeks' gestation are placed on the radiant warmer on top of a heating pad, are covered with clear plastic wrap or a plastic bag from the neck down, and wear a soft cloth hat to help prevent heat loss.

Breathing

Most babies make some crying efforts in the first minute after birth. The neonatal team may encourage breathing by gently rubbing the baby's back. If your baby does not breathe in a few moments, is too weak to breathe regularly, or has a slow heart rate (*pulse*), the neonatal team will place a soft mask over the baby's nose and mouth and use a mechanical device to inflate the baby's lungs and assist breathing. This is called *positive-pressure ventilation* (*PPV*). Most babies will respond with an increasing heart rate, and most will begin breathing on their own.

A neonatal team member places a face mask firmly over the baby's nose and mouth and uses a resuscitation bag to deliver air/oxygen into the baby's lungs. Positive-pressure ventilation is necessary when the baby is not breathing or when the baby's heart rate is slow.

Courtesy of Gigi O'Dea.

If your baby is breathing and has a normal heart rate but appears to be working hard to breathe, the team may place a soft mask over the baby's mouth and nose and use a mechanical device to maintain a steady stream of air pressure in the lungs. This constant air pressure is called *continuous positive airway pressure* (*CPAP*) and helps to keep the tiny air sacs in the baby's lungs (*alveoli*) open between breaths. This can make breathing easier. Continuous positive airway pressure can also be given using tubing with short prongs that fit into the baby's nose or a special mask placed over the baby's nose. You may notice a bubbling bottle of water at the end of the tubing that supplies the air pressure.

Meridith is breathing on her own but needs CPAP to make her breathing easier.

Oxygen

The air we breathe (called room air) contains about 21% oxygen. During resuscitation, your baby's need for additional oxygen is monitored with *pulse oximetry*. A *pulse oximeter* is a device that wraps around the baby's hand or wrist to measure the amount of oxygen attached to the RBCs. The device shines a small red light through the skin and is painless. The pulse oximeter displays a number called *oxygen saturation* (abbreviated as SpO_2). Based on your baby's age in minutes, a special chart is used to identify the oxygen saturation *target* and guide the administration of additional oxygen.

Intubation

If your baby does not begin to breathe after several minutes of assistance or if the heart rate remains low, a thin plastic tube may be placed in the baby's mouth and advanced into the windpipe (*trachea*). This process is called *intubation,* and the tube is called an *endotracheal tube.* An endotracheal tube provides a direct route to your baby's lungs and allows the team to help your baby breathe more effectively. The tube can be attached to a resuscitation device that temporarily provides additional air pressure and oxygen or to a respirator (*ventilator*) for more prolonged assistance with breathing. Because the tube is positioned between your baby's vocal cords, your baby will not be able to make crying noises while the tube is in place. When your baby no longer needs the endotracheal tube, it is removed. This is called *extubation.*

Eliana, born extremely preterm at 23 weeks' gestation, required intubation at birth.

This is **Auggie** at 24 weeks of gestation and just minutes old. He wears a soft cloth hat and is wrapped in plastic to maintain his body temperature. The care provider holds the inflated bag and delivers gentle breaths into his lungs through his endotracheal tube.

Surfactant

Surfactant is a soapy substance usually produced by lung cells that helps to keep the lungs inflated. Production of surfactant begins at about 24 weeks of gestation but is not well developed until about 36 weeks of gestation. Some preterm babies will have breathing difficulty because they do not have enough surfactant in their lungs. Giving corticosteroids to the pregnant person before the birth (*antenatal steroids*) speeds up the production of surfactant in the

baby's lungs. Many preterm newborns will improve with CPAP only, but others will need to receive additional surfactant after birth. Surfactant can be instilled into the baby's lungs through an endotracheal tube or thin catheter.

If your baby will be born preterm, ask the neonatologist what you can expect regarding the use of CPAP and surfactant administration in the delivery room or NICU (see Chapter 5).

Abel, born at 22 weeks and 5 days, also required intubation. He has a blood pressure cuff around his left arm, a pulse oximeter sensor on his right wrist, and umbilical catheters visible on his abdomen. The plastic wrap helps maintain his body temperature.

Chest Compressions, Emergency Umbilical Vein Catheter, and Epinephrine

In rare cases, a baby is so seriously ill that the heart rate remains very low and does not improve with breaths given through an endotracheal tube. When this happens, *chest compressions* (pushing on the baby's chest) and a lifesaving medication called *epinephrine* (also called *adrenaline*) may be needed. A thin tube called an emergency *umbilical vein catheter (UVC)* can be placed quickly into the large vein in the umbilical cord, allowing the neonatal team to administer medications and fluids directly into the baby's bloodstream. A UVC may also be placed after resuscitation if your baby needs an IV for more than a few days (see Chapter 3).

Apgar Score

At 1 minute of age, again at 5 minutes, and every 5 minutes thereafter until babies are stabilized, they are assessed and given a numerical score to reflect their general condition. This scoring system was created by a physician, Dr. Virginia Apgar, in the 1950s and is named after her. *Apgar scores* give the neonatal team an indication of the baby's overall condition and the transition to life outside of the uterus. The score is used to standardize the way health care professionals describe a baby's transition after birth but it does not predict your baby's IQ or future intelligence.

To determine your baby's Apgar score, the health care team assesses 5 categories: heart rate, breathing, color, muscle tone, and reflexes. Babies are assigned a score of 0, 1, or 2 in each category, with 0 indicating absent or very depressed responses and 2 indicating very active responses. The Apgar score is the total of the 5 numbers. When the baby receives assistance at birth, an expanded Apgar score may be used (see the Expanded Apgar Score chart in the Appendix) to document the kind of help the baby was receiving when the score was assigned in each category.

Few babies receive an Apgar score of 10 because a baby's hands and feet normally remain blue for a while. A full-term, healthy, crying baby usually receives an Apgar score of 8 or 9. Keep in mind, however, that very preterm babies receive lower Apgar scores than full-term newborns simply because they are immature and unable to respond with loud crying and strong muscle tone.

Transferring the Newborn to Another Hospital

Babies who require specialized care not offered at their birth hospital will be transferred to a NICU at another hospital (*neonatal transport*). Your baby's medical provider will contact the NICU and arrange the transfer. Depending on the condition of your baby and the distance between the baby's birth hospital and the NICU, your baby may be transported by ambulance, helicopter, or airplane.

Newborn Transport Preparation

A specially trained neonatal transport team will prepare your baby for the trip and continue intensive care while traveling to the NICU. Your baby will be inside a transport incubator, designed to provide warmth while allowing immediate access for any care needed during transport.

If possible, before leaving the birth hospital, the transport team will bring your baby to your hospital room. Separation from your new baby is difficult. If still recovering from surgery and anesthesia, the birthing parent may not even remember seeing the baby before transport. Some families take photos using their phone or camera before the baby leaves. Even if your baby is not critically ill, separation is frightening and increases your stress.

Before the transport team leaves, be sure you have the NICU phone number, know how you will be informed when your baby arrives at the NICU, and know how to call the NICU so that you can check on your baby whenever you wish. If the breastfeeding parent has pumped and stored breast milk, talk with the transport team about sending it with them to support your baby's oral care and initiation of feeding when ready.

> " Going through this journey was overwhelming at first and we couldn't have done it without a plan. We had another daughter who was 9 at the time so we had to figure out how to balance normal life with NICU life. We would drop her off at school, then drive about an hour to the hospital in time for rounds to see Eliana's care team, ask questions if we needed to, and learn what the plan of action was for that day. On the weekends, we decided we would stay overnight at the hospital and have our 9-year-old daughter take turns with family and friends with fun sleepovers. "

*Sophany, mother of **Eliana***

Staying in Touch

A member of the NICU team at the receiving hospital will call after your baby arrives and update you on your baby's condition. If you do not understand what you are told, ask the NICU provider to explain the situation in words you can understand. The doctor and nurse at your birth hospital may also help explain your baby's condition.

If the NICU is far from the hospital, you and your partner may be faced with the additional challenge of figuring out how to be in 2 places at once. Long-distance transport is especially difficult if you have other children at home who need your attention.

Ask your hospital discharge planner or social worker about hotels near your baby, and try to spend some time with your baby as soon as possible. If you must return home right away, ask about the system for staying in touch with the NICU. Your baby's NICU doctor or nurse may set up a time to call you every day and tell you about your baby's progress, and you will be given the phone number to call whenever you wish. Some NICUs will send or email you a photograph and short note "from your baby" each week. Some NICUs have a video system so you can see your baby on your laptop, tablet, or smartphone.

Sorting It Out

To process and understand their birthing experience, many new parents feel the need to tell and retell the story of labor and birth. This recounting of events can be especially important for parents of a baby who needs intensive care. When your baby's birth becomes a series of unexpected events, the whole experience may take on a dreamlike quality, making it hard for you to know what actually happened. Until the experience becomes real to you, coping with the challenges of NICU parenting can be difficult.

Each parent may have a slightly different version of what happened and feel varying levels of responsibility and powerlessness. Parents of babies in the NICU may feel a sense of loss and failure. They may feel torn in multiple directions trying to meet the needs of their other children, family members, sick newborn (or newborns), and partner. The NICU staff can be a great help as you search for answers to your questions and sort out your feelings. Once you begin to understand what happened and can place the events in order, you can begin to move ahead. This will not happen all at once or at the same time for everyone. Allow yourself time for personal recovery and take advantage of supportive people who will listen to your story. You will also discover that NICU parents often find support by sharing their experiences with other NICU parents. Your ability to cope will grow over time as you learn about the resources available and gain the strength to move forward.

> **"** The reality of what was happening did not kick in when the contractions did. It didn't even kick in when I delivered in the operating room and my son was whisked off. It was all so surreal and what I had envisioned for the moments after birth was not at all what I had experienced. That was hard to accept. Finally, the reality hit me and I had to accept the fact that other people were going to help my baby survive. **"**
>
> *Marnie, mother of **Kellan***

Eliana

Born at 23 weeks

We had Eliana through IVF after years and years of failed pregnancy attempts, after an adoption through foster care, and after finally getting pregnant but then losing our son at 17 weeks. The pregnancy with Eliana went well up until about 20 weeks, when I started having complications. My cervix was shortening, and it was too late to do any interventions. We did not want to lose our baby again. Our faith in God carried us through it all. We prayed and did everything we could to delay my labor.

Eliana, 10 days old, enjoys kangaroo care with her father.

At exactly 23 weeks, in fall of 2019, Eliana was born weighing just under 1½ pounds. She was on a ventilator right away since her lungs were not fully developed. Everything happened so fast. Being first time parents to a newborn is already scary but we were first time parents to a baby born at 23 weeks. With so many unknowns, we were terrified.

The doctors and nurses were very helpful in explaining everything to us in detail, but it was all still so overwhelming. We were nervous to hold and touch her with all the wires and cords connected to her and she looked so tiny and fragile. The nurses encouraged us and talked us through everything, giving us confidence. We made sure we did kangaroo care every day with Eliana because we didn't know what else to do. There's just something about that skin-on-skin contact that connects you as a parent to your child. The nurses truly empowered us and taught us how to be parents to our micropreemie.

Going through this journey was overwhelming at first and we couldn't have done it without a plan. We had another daughter who was 9 at the time so we had to figure out how to balance normal life with NICU life. We would drop her off at school, then drive about an hour to the hospital in time for rounds to see Eliana's care team, ask questions if we needed to, and learn what the plan of action was for that day. The nurses were always there to go into detail about the care plan if we missed rounds or if we did not fully understand everything. We would leave around 4 pm so we could beat

Eliana at age 3 weeks.

Eliana is ready to go home at age 3 months.

the traffic and pick our daughter up from the after-school program, have dinner, help with homework and spend some time with her, then do it all over again. On the weekends, we decided we would stay overnight at the hospital and have our 9-year-old daughter take turns with family and friends with fun sleepovers. This routine worked for our family and may not have worked for everyone, but I would say, make a plan, be consistent, and stick with it.

Eliana was a fighter from the start. She was feisty and fierce but still had to go through one surgery to close her PDA (an opening between the aorta and the pulmonary artery). It wasn't closing on its own and because of that, it was hard for her to feed and grow, she was dependent on supplemental oxygen, and had a hard time breathing on her own. Because she was on a ventilator longer than the doctors wanted, we tried a couple of different therapies. Eventually, she was able to switch to CPAP, and finally to a nasal cannula.

In March 2020, we were able to take her home! She weighed about 5 pounds and was doing great. We took her home on a low flow oxygen tank and a feeding tube because she wasn't fully feeding on her own quite yet. We were lucky to come home about a week before everything shut down due to COVID, and this was a total blessing! Within a couple of days, she pulled out her feeding tube while sleeping and she never needed it after that. Over the next 3 months, we were able to wean her off her oxygen and she has been doing amazingly ever since!

Eliana is now 2 years old and is growing, running, climbing, talking, learning, and definitely as feisty as ever! Since we've been home, we've had many appointments with the neonatologist, ophthalmologist, physical therapist, occupational therapist, and a speech therapist, all working together to get her where she needs to be.

At age 2, Eliana loves to help with the cooking.

Having a preemie in the NICU was probably one of the hardest things we've ever had to go through, but truly worth all the tears, all the driving back and forth, all the back pains from sleeping on the hospital couch, all the meals we had to eat at the hospital, and all the questions we had to ask many times over because we didn't understand. Looking back, it really didn't seem like 100 days in the NICU because we made lasting friendships, we have our miracle baby, and we have an incredible story to tell.

Sophany and Mike, parents of Eliana

Eliana's family in 2022: Alliyah, Mike, Sophany, and Eliana

Lucy

Born at 29 weeks
. . . .

I was just entering my third trimester and my pregnancy had gone relatively smoothly. I had a little bit of spotting over the weekend at 29 weeks and went to the hospital and checked out fine. Matt and I went to our routine prenatal appointment the next morning and I again checked out fine and was cleared to fly on a business trip the next day.

Matt and I said good-bye and I went to work. About 30 minutes later, my water broke. A friend drove me to the hospital and Matt met me there. They tried to slow things down, but Lucy had other ideas and was born at 5:39 that night. During her birth, Lucy's heart rate dropped dramatically and I was scared that we were going to lose her. It was overwhelming. She was 3 pounds 13 ounces and had a head full of hair. She was absolutely perfect.

Lucy makes progress in the NICU.

During our NICU stay, Lucy had a lot of trouble with "events" (apnea and bradycardia), particularly with any attempts at feeding. She could not handle breastfeeding and struggled with bottles until right before our discharge day. It took us a few weeks to settle into a NICU routine, but once we found our rhythm and schedule, things became a lot easier and fun at times. The NICU is full of amazing people who dedicate their lives to treating and helping the tiniest of humans.

Our NICU stay was 71 days and we went home 3 days before my due date. Any NICU stay, no matter if it is a few hours or several months, is difficult and scary for parents. It is usually not part of your plan or what you envision for the start of your child's life and it is a surreal place that most people know very little about. Also, in the beginning, I struggled with a lot of guilt about why she came early and blamed myself for her early birth and struggles in the NICU.

Lucy next to her preemie pajamas.

Lucy with her parents.

It is often hard to believe this girl was the little 3-pound preemie we fell in love with! Today, Lucy is toddling around our house, laughing and smiling and carrying on. It is so fun seeing her learn things on a daily basis and her vocabulary (both verbal and sign language) is exploding right now. In the last couple weeks, she's started nodding "yes" to things. She's become obsessed with cats (pictures of cats, actual cats, drawings of cats, even abstract illustrations of cats), which is particularly odd since we don't have a cat. Lucy also loves watermelon, books, baths, opening and closing everything, and all music.

Lucy is caring, gentle, and shy. In short, she's a fun little person, and she's awesome to spend time with. Looking back, I love that we got to know her when she was so little and got to see how she has grown and overcome so much since that day we met her. **Read more about Lucy in "Where Are They Now?" in the Appendix.**

Kate and Matt, parents of Lucy

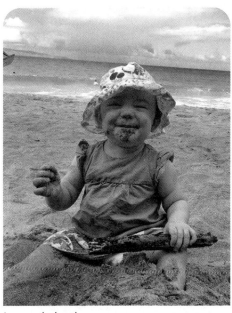

Lucy on the beach.

CHAPTER 2

The NICU Journey Begins

> Everything happened so fast.
> Being first-time parents to a
> newborn is already scary,
> but we were first-time parents
> to a baby born at 23 weeks.
> With so many unknowns,
> we were terrified.
>
> *Sophany and Mike, parents of **Eliana***

The moment of birth is usually a triumphant celebration. Not only have you made it through labor and birth, you've welcomed into your family a new little person who carries your dreams for the future. When things don't go as expected, you face a more stressful beginning than most parents. You and your partner need to deal with the feelings of loss that accompany the birth of a sick or preterm baby. For most parents, the neonatal intensive care unit (NICU) is a new world of medical vocabulary and technology that may, at first, seem overwhelming.

First Steps

Each neonatal intensive care nursery has its own routines, but most share certain common priorities when a new baby is admitted. Here are explanations of typical activities during NICU admission.

The Admission Process

Between birth and your baby's arrival in the NICU, many things happen at once. Doctors, nurses, and respiratory therapists will stabilize your baby's condition; begin diagnostic tests, if necessary; and establish the immediate care plan. Priorities in the first hour include making sure your baby is breathing well and keeping your baby's oxygen saturation, heart rate, blood pressure, blood sugar, and body temperature all within normal levels. Your baby is weighed, a hospital identification bracelet is placed on the baby's wrist or foot, an injection of vitamin K is given to prevent potential bleeding difficulties, and antibiotic ointment is placed in your baby's eyes to prevent infection. During the first hour, the NICU team may perform special procedures to assist your infant's breathing, obtain blood samples for tests, and insert thin tubes (*catheters*) into veins or arteries to give medications and fluids. While the team is performing these procedures, you may not be able to see your baby because the baby may be under sterile drapes. Additional routine procedures, such as measuring the baby's length and obtaining footprints, may be delayed until your newborn's condition is more stable.

First Trip to the NICU

Your NICU team will be very busy during the first hour of your baby's arrival. If you must wait to see your infant, minutes may seem like hours. Within the first 60 minutes, a member of the team should be available to give you and your partner an update, describe what procedures have been completed, and explain the initial plan. The team members will do everything they can to bring you to your baby's bedside as quickly as possible. They know it is important for parents to see their newborns, touch them, talk to them, and take photos.

The experience of becoming a NICU parent is different for everyone. Parents often describe their first day or two in the NICU as "foggy and dreamlike." You may feel helpless and wonder how you will ever be able to participate in your baby's care, especially if your baby is transported to the NICU from another hospital. Most NICU nurses and physicians are good at keeping parents informed. They will probably tell you more than you can understand at first, so don't worry if things seem unclear. Very soon, you will begin to understand your newborn's problems, get to know your NICU team, understand their routines, and begin to participate as partners in your baby's care.

When you and your partner first arrive in the NICU, and every time you come after that, you will need to clean your hands thoroughly either at a sink or with alcohol-based hand sanitizer. Most likely, the staff will also have an alcohol-based hand sanitizer at your baby's bedside and ask you to use it every time before and after you touch your baby.

Special Considerations for Birthing Parents

Depending on the circumstances at birth, your baby may have been taken immediately to the NICU, without you getting as much as a glimpse of this new member of your family. If you experienced a high-risk birth or an emergency cesarean delivery, you may have had general anesthesia and your partner or support person may not have been able to attend the birth. You may see your new baby for the first time in the NICU.

These are some things you can do to make the most of your first moments in the NICU.

▸ If you are exhausted, consider taking a short nap before going to the NICU.

▸ Write down questions you want to ask.

▸ Eat something if it has been a while since you had a meal.

▸ Consider using a pump or hand expressing breast milk to prepare for your baby's nutritional needs. Ask your nurse or lactation specialist for help.

▸ If your partner or support person has already been to the NICU, talk about what you can expect to see and how your baby is doing.

▸ Use the bathroom before going to the NICU. People who have just given birth need to urinate frequently, and the parent restroom may be outside of the NICU.

▸ If you have just given birth, consider going to the NICU by wheelchair. You may feel energized after delivery, but a long walk to the NICU will drain your energy and cut your visit short. The wheelchair is a good way to save energy and it's handy if you feel light-headed and need to sit down.

Ellie's parents visit the NICU for the first time. Melissa is supported by a person in front, who holds her arm, and by her husband who stands behind her. The nurse at the warmer helps Melissa touch her baby.

> ❝ Any NICU stay, no matter if it is a few hours or several months, is difficult and scary for parents. It is usually not part of your plan or what you envision for the start of your child's life, and it is a surreal place that most people know very little about. ❞
>
> *Matt, father of* **Lucy**

Your Baby's Care Team

Every NICU has its own team structure and mixture of team players. Each member of the group is equally important and all team members work together to care for your baby. You may meet some of these people before, during, or after admission to the NICU.

Nursing Team

Neonatal Intensive Care Unit (NICU) Nurse

A NICU nurse is a registered nurse (RN) and provides most of the moment-to-moment bedside care for your baby. A NICU nurse has special training in the care of newborns requiring intensive care and their families.

The health care professionals in the neonatal intensive care unit use every opportunity to teach you about your baby's care. This nurse answers a mother's questions and encourages her to talk to her baby.

Courtesy of Seattle Children's Hospital.

The NICU nurse participates in making the daily care plan with the NICU physician, neonatal nurse practitioner (NNP), or physician assistant (PA) based on their assessment of your baby's condition. The nurse carries out the medical team's orders and notifies them of any changes in your baby's status. In addition, NICU nurses play a key role in parent education and discharge planning.

> " Thirty-seven days of ups and downs but a lifetime ahead of being grateful for the knowledge of the people around us. "
>
> *Marnie, mother of* **Kellan**

Nursing Education and Leadership

The nursing team is supported by a *charge nurse* who oversees the nursing operations for each nursing shift. Behind the scenes, most NICUs also have a NICU nurse manager who provides supervision and leadership for all of the nursing staff. Many NICUs have a clinical nurse specialist or a nurse educator who serves as a clinical expert, leads staff education, and may lead nursing research, quality improvement, and program development.

Medical Team

Your baby may receive care from more medical professionals than you have encountered in your entire life. In every NICU, a member of the medical team is usually present in the NICU 24 hours a day and a supervising physician is always on call for that unit.

Neonatologist

A neonatologist is a physician who specializes in the diagnosis and treatment of sick newborns. The neonatologist has completed medical school, residency training in pediatrics, and then additional training in neonatology. In many NICUs, the neonatologist is the lead physician, referred to as the *attending physician,* and directs the medical care of your baby. The attending physician is responsible for supervising the other members of the medical team.

Fellow

A neonatology fellow is a physician who has completed medical school and pediatric residency and is training to become a neonatologist. The fellow works with the attending physician to develop the care plan and supervise the other members of the team.

Resident

A resident is a physician who has graduated from medical school and is completing additional training in a medical specialty (for example, pediatrics, obstetrics, family medicine). The resident assesses your newborn daily and plans the medical care with supervision from the attending physician and fellow.

Pediatric Hospitalist

A pediatric hospitalist is a physician who has completed pediatric residency and has focused their practice on the care of babies and children in the hospital.

Neonatal Nurse Practitioner

An NNP, also called an advanced registered nurse practitioner (ARNP), is not a doctor but is part of the medical team. An NNP is an RN who has completed advanced training in the care and treatment of sick newborns. An NNP has a master's degree in nursing, and some have a doctoral degree. The NNP works in collaboration with other members of the medical team to examine newborns, make a diagnosis, and develop the treatment plan.

Physician Assistant

A PA is a licensed medical professional who works under the supervision of a physician to examine newborns, make a diagnosis, and develop the treatment plan.

More Doctors in the House

Your baby's medical team may call on other pediatric specialists to assist them in providing care for your baby. These consultants may be present in your hospital or available on an intermittent basis or by telephone.

- **Cardiac surgeon:** specializes in performing surgery on the heart
- **Cardiologist:** specializes in diagnosis and treatment of heart problems
- **Gastroenterologist:** specializes in diagnosis and treatment of stomach and intestinal problems
- **Geneticist:** specializes in diagnosis and treatment of genetic syndromes and congenital anomalies.
- **Hematologist:** specializes in diagnosis and treatment of blood problems
- **Nephrologist:** specializes in diagnosis and medical treatment of kidney problems
- **Neurologist:** specializes in diagnosis and treatment of the nervous system (brain, spinal cord, nerves)
- **Neurosurgeon:** specializes in surgery of the brain and nervous system
- **Pediatric surgeon:** specializes in performing surgery on newborns and children
- **Pulmonologist:** specializes in diagnosis and treatment of lung conditions and breathing problems
- **Urologist:** specializes in surgical treatment of the kidneys and urinary tract

> ❝ The nurses were always there to go into detail about the care plan if we missed rounds or if we did not fully understand everything. Do not be afraid to ask! Everyone was always willing to talk and so very helpful! ❞
>
> *Sophany, mother of **Eliana***

Support Team

It takes a village to raise a child, and there exists a village in the NICU to support the medical team, nursing team, and your baby. Again, each NICU may have some or all of these team members, and not every baby will require the services of these team members.

▶ **Case manager/discharge planner:** Follows your baby's hospital course, assists with insurance issues, and helps to organize details for your baby's discharge.

▶ **Chaplain:** Provides spiritual comfort or guidance, if requested.

▶ **Financial or billing representative:** Answers questions about your hospital bills, helps you submit your bills to the appropriate agencies for payment, and sets up a payment plan, if needed.

▶ **Lactation specialist:** Supports and educates NICU staff, parents, and babies regarding lactation.

▶ **Dietitian:** Analyzes your baby's energy and nutritional needs and makes suggestions about intravenous nutrition and additives for breast milk or formula.

▶ **Peer parent support person (may be called parent-to-parent support, family support, or parent host):** Former NICU parent trained to provide support and a listening ear to parents who have little or no NICU experience.

▶ **Pharmacist:** Helps ensure the safety of medications and intravenous nutrition for newborns.

▶ **Psychologist:** A trained mental health professional who specializes in helping parents cope with stressful situations, difficult emotions, grief, depression, or anxiety.

▶ **Respiratory therapist:** Specializes in treating problems of the respiratory system. Works under the direction of medical professionals to evaluate and monitor lung function and manage equipment and devices for breathing treatments.

▶ **Social worker:** Helps families cope with stress, deal with financial concerns, use hospital and community resources, and prepare for discharge to home.

- **Students in health care profession programs:** Includes students of nursing, medicine, respiratory therapy, and others. Students do not perform complex procedures and are highly supervised while learning in the NICU.
- **Therapists:** Occupational, physical, speech, massage, and music therapists all have special skills to help your baby's neurologic and physical development.
- **Unit coordinator:** Manages the flow of people, paper, and information into and out of the NICU. Also called a unit secretary, patient services coordinator, or unit clerk.
- **Still more people:** Other personnel include laboratory technicians (trained to obtain blood samples), x-ray technicians, ultrasound technicians, team members who help keep bedside supplies stocked, and housekeepers. Sometimes, staff members are cross-trained, which means they can work in more than one hospital unit and help nurses by taking routine vital signs and transporting patients to different areas of the hospital.

Have We Met Before?

It is possible that in a large children's hospital or regional medical center, you may meet a new physician every week! No wonder you're confused about who is caring for your baby. Until you become familiar with the system, introduce yourself every time you see an unfamiliar face, and never feel shy about asking a team member to identify their role on the team. It is your right to know who is caring for your baby. Some NICUs may have an information board or an area where the team's pictures and role descriptions are posted to help you recognize the team.

> " Many of the people who took care of Lucy became our friends. These people will laugh with you, cry with you, teach you to parent, empower you, and cheer you on when you walk out those doors on discharge day. They are there for some of the hardest things you'll ever experience, and they're fantastic. "

*Kate and Matt, parents of **Lucy***

Rhythms and Schedules

Scheduling in the NICU is designed to achieve around-the-clock medical and nursing care for patients. Members of the nursing and medical teams work a variety of shifts to ensure that appropriate health care professionals are available in the NICU 24 hours a day.

> 66 My first trip to the NICU was a bit unique. I couldn't leave my hospital bed for 24 hours after giving birth, and I was aching to see my baby. My fabulous nurse rolled my entire hospital bed up to the NICU and I held Logan's hand for the first time! 99
>
> *Christina, mother of **Logan***

NICU Nurses

Some NICUs use a system called *primary nursing* to allow nurses to get to know specific patients and care for them when they are at work. This system allows a small number of nurses to become most familiar with you and your baby's individual needs. In any case, the nurses who care for your baby are knowledgeable about the plan of care and are interested in helping you learn about your baby and prepare for discharge.

NICU Medical Staff

The members of your baby's medical team may have other responsibilities in the hospital and may change assignments weekly, biweekly, or monthly. These assignment changes are called *rotations*. This means that over time, you may have a different group of doctors assigned to your baby's care. Neonatal intensive care units use multiple systems to ensure uninterrupted quality care for your baby through these shift changes and rotations.

To find a balance between continuity of care and ensuring your baby's medical team is appropriately rested, most hospital systems have implemented *duty-hour restrictions* for medical professionals. This means the medical team often shares overnight and weekend *on-call* responsibilities so no one works an excessive number of hours. Hospitals use a variety of different plans to divide work among medical professionals. If you have questions during the night or weekend, you may meet with the medical professionals who are on call for your baby's team. During your stay in the NICU, you will gradually become familiar with all members of the medical team.

The Information Playbook

The trust between you and your baby's team is built on communication. Open, direct, and honest communication is vital for families with a baby in the NICU.

Patient Rounds

Many people with different kinds of expertise are dedicated to caring for your baby. How do all these people coordinate their ideas and plans? The most common and time-honored tradition of medical team communication is called *patient rounds*. This is when doctors, NNPs, PAs, hospitalists, nurses, respiratory therapists, dietitians, pharmacists, and others involved in your baby's care get together to review the previous day's events and make a plan for the next few days. The purpose of patient rounds is to make sure that information is shared accurately, the plan of care moves forward in a coordinated way, and everyone is working toward the day when your baby can go home.

Most NICUs welcome parents to rounds. You are important members of your baby's care team. Your observations of your baby are important to the team's understanding of how your baby is doing. When you share your observations and ideas with the care team during rounds and participate in making decisions, you help the team provide the best care possible for your baby.

> " Each morning, the doctors and nurses would go room by room talking through each case and planning goals for the day. We quickly found their meetings were filled with lots of useful information, including what they were planning on doing with Ellie for the day, new information about what they thought had happened to her, and anything else pertinent for the day or week. "
>
> *Melissa, mother of **Ellie***

These parents are participating in rounds. Sharing your observations about your baby is very important to providing the best possible care.

Courtesy of George A. Little, MD, FAAP.

The Care Plan

By understanding your baby's care plan, you may better understand daily routines and be able to recognize milestones in your baby's NICU experience.

The care plan guides how and when things are done. It often describes topics like what kind of breathing support your baby will receive, how additional oxygen and breathing support will be adjusted, when and how to begin or increase feedings, and when your baby is ready to graduate from an incubator to a crib. These plans are customized to meet your baby's own medical needs.

It is also important to realize that care plans change. Care plans must be flexible; they depend on your baby's response to treatments and overall condition. Ask often for an update on the care plan. If the plan has changed, you may want to ask, "What is different now that caused this change in the plan?" If your baby's condition has changed but the care plan has not, you may ask, "Why hasn't the plan changed even though my baby hasn't [or has] gotten better?" Asking these simple questions allows you to stay informed, prepare for changes, and participate in your baby's care.

Your baby's medical problems are probably new to you; however, your baby's problems may be common in the NICU. Many NICUs have developed care maps, clinical pathways, or discharge readiness milestones that show the usual path of a common diagnosis. For example, the clinical pathway for a healthy 34 weeks' gestation preterm baby shows what to expect at first and what milestones the baby has to achieve before going home. Seeing on a list or road map what needs to happen may help you understand the road you and your baby are traveling and the path toward going home.

> "Advocate, advocate, advocate. You know your baby best and if you see something that isn't right, say something."
>
> *Mary Ellen, mother of **Meridith***

Learning Common Terms, Phrases, and Problems

Learning the words and concepts you hear about in rounds and in the NICU can help you feel more relaxed and comfortable. For efficiency, members of your baby's care team may talk to each other using medical abbreviations and terminology, and sometimes they may forget to translate these terms for you. You are not expected to be a medical expert and should never feel like you have to do homework to know about your baby's care. Do not hesitate to ask your doctor or nurse for explanations. Most NICU providers really enjoy talking with parents and explaining the treatment plan.

Some parents feel more comfortable learning about NICU terms, phrases, and problems at their own pace. Reading this book will help. Your NICU may also have a parent support program to help you learn about the NICU experience. Talking with other parents who have shared this experience may also be helpful. Some NICUs have a parent resource center with books about babies in the NICU and internet access to find information. Be cautious about the information you read on the internet or social media. Anyone can post information, but not all of it is accurate. Ask for website recommendations from a parent educator, a family resource center specialist, or a member of your baby's NICU team. Additionally, although social media can connect you with other families who had newborns in the NICU, not all of their experiences may relate to your infant and family. Many NICUs have specific social media groups that you may wish to join as you build your NICU community. The more you understand, the better you can support your baby.

> ❝ During our weeks in the NICU, I picked up the terminology. I asked questions and I made sure that I understood what was happening at any given time and what the next steps were. Feeling educated helped me feel in control. ❞
>
> *Marnie, mother of* **Kellan**

Making Sure You Get the Information You Want and Need

"What if?" Questions

All too often, parents do not ask the "what if?" questions and then become frustrated because their questions have not been addressed. Asking "what if?" questions can make you better informed about the treatment, procedure, or medication in question.

▸ "What if this treatment doesn't work?"

▸ "What if we decide against surgery?"

▸ "What if this problem gets worse?"

Keep in mind that, at times, a perfect answer doesn't exist. Sometimes, the approach to the same problem will vary between hospitals and between health professionals within the same hospital. Most often, neither approach is wrong. Sometimes, the treatment that seemed to work well at one point in your baby's NICU stay doesn't work as well at another time, and your baby's team will have to try a different approach. While the knowledge and expertise to care for babies keep improving, there are times when a decision must be made by carefully weighing the risks and benefits and then choosing what seems to be the best course at that time.

What Kind of Information Do You Want?

When you ask your baby's doctor or nurse, "How is my baby today?" you may think it's a simple question, but NICU staff may have difficulty knowing how much and what type of information you expect. Some parents want specific clinical information, such as laboratory results and ventilator settings. Other parents prefer more general information, such as how well their baby slept or whether their baby is tolerating feedings.

Tell your baby's care providers about the type of information you want, how you'd like to receive it, and when you want to know it. Tell them the best way and time to reach you. Give them some examples. Do you want to be called immediately with test results regardless of the time of day, or can you wait to be told when you visit? Is there a time of day when you shouldn't be called? Do you want to know only the unusual test results, or do you want to know most test results? Be honest with the NICU staff. Don't expect your baby's caregivers to read your mind. Your preferences for information will likely change over time, so remember to update your baby's care team about what you want to know and when.

Scheduling Time With the People You Want to See

As you will learn, schedules in the NICU may not always be consistent. The team may usually make rounds at the same time each morning, but then an emergency in the delivery room or with another baby in the NICU changes their schedule. Even if you have been told the neo-natologist is usually in the unit at a certain time, do not plan to "catch" the physician for a lengthy chat during patient rounds. A more effective approach is to schedule a time to discuss your baby's progress in person or by telephone. This gives the people involved time to review and organize the most up-to-date information about your baby's care. A scheduled time also decreases the chance you will be interrupted while discussing your questions and concerns.

Care Conferences/Family Meetings

Your baby's team may schedule what is called a *care conference* or *family meeting* for you, or you may request one. These meetings help familiarize you with team members you may not see daily. Sitting down and talking with several team members (for example, nursing team, medical team, respiratory therapists, medical subspecialty and surgical consulting doctors, social workers) gives you the chance to ask questions of different team members at once, get updates on any big changes in your baby's plan of care, and learn what progress the team is hoping to see from your baby.

When the Unexpected Happens

Sometimes, even the most skilled care team can make a mistake. Staying involved in your baby's care and treatment plan is one way to help the team avoid errors. If you are at your baby's bedside and see something that doesn't seem right, alert your baby's nurse or another member of the NICU team.

Give Yourself Some Time

Each NICU is a community with its own customs, language, codes of behavior, and habits. You are becoming part of this new community while your whole world has been turned upside down. You will need some time to adjust to this new environment.

After your first NICU visits, you may feel overwhelmed and out of place. In time, you will get to know the people caring for your baby and what they do. With patience, you will develop valuable relationships with them. These are the first important steps toward active involvement in your baby's care.

Isaac
&
Eliza

Born at 27 weeks, 3 days

It was a regular August weekend for our family. We had homemade pizza and some fruit for linner (late lunch and early dinner). We ended our day relaxing and getting ready for the next day of work for us and school for Ethan.

Overnight we had very heavy rain and a thunderstorm. I woke up in the middle of the night feeling odd and anxious. I called the university OB-GYN Triage line. They told me to take a nice warm shower and relax and everything would be okay. I followed their instructions and went back to sleep but inside my gut I knew something wasn't right with the twins.

In the morning, I woke up with heavy bleeding. We rushed to the hospital where doctors tried to figure out what was going on. Suddenly, I felt a big gush of water. I was exactly 25 weeks pregnant.

We knew at that point my water had broken, but we did not know if it was for both babies or just one. The first 24 hours was a big dark hole. I do not recall anything except talking to the NICU doctor, who went over statistics of survival for both and/or one baby. She connected us to a NICU Parent Host who gave us a NICU tour the next day. After many ultrasounds, we learned that only Isaac's water had broken, so we would keep the pregnancy going as long as possible with minimal movement and major hospital bedrest.

Overnight our perfectly healthy pregnancy changed to a high-risk pregnancy with the possibility of losing both babies. It was the hardest 2 weeks and 3 days of my life because I had no idea what the outcome would be. I wanted to avoid going into labor because I didn't want to face the reality of making difficult choices about the survival of Baby A, Baby B or both, or me. At that point, I tried to stay in the present by crossing off the date on the calendar every 24 hours. I kept my pregnancy going until I was 27 weeks and 3 days when I had to have an emergency C-section. Isaac was born weighing 2 pounds 0.8 ounce and Eliza was a little bigger, weighing in at 2 pounds 3 ounces.

The NICU team took our babies away immediately and started working to make sure they had the highest chance of survival. I was so drained and shocked that it took me a long time to recover well enough after surgery to move to my own room. I recall being in a lot of pain and refusing to see the babies because I did not know what the outcome would be.

Parina holds the twins together for the first time.

The next day, the lactation consultant came to my room and asked me to start pumping. I was in a very deep depression at that point. I had given up all hope about our babies and all I wanted to do was cuddle up in a corner of the room. I was convinced that they were not going to make it out of the NICU. I still remember the one thing that changed my perspective on the whole situation. She said, "Hun, you have no control over the outcome of your babies or even what will happen in the next 30 minutes or tomorrow. You *do have one thing you can control,* which is pumping or trying to pump milk for your babies. Why do you want to give up that control?" I started pumping and decided to take my milk to my babies almost 72 hours after birth.

Isaac and Eliza touch hands for balance as they learn to sit.

I decided to see Isaac first. He was tiny and covered with so many wires and tubes. Preemie diapers looked so big on him. All I could do was watch him take every breath and his entire body was moving. I could see all of his ribs through his skin. Such a tiny hand and leg but a full head of black hair.

The next day I built all my strength and went to the NICU to see Eliza. At that point, Eliza had been in room air for over an hour and that was a big milestone. I looked at her sleeping helplessly, her skin so wrinkled. The nurse told me the twins were doing amazingly despite their size, weight, and prematurity.

I decided to spend a day in the NICU after my own discharge. It was the scariest experience. They would both stop breathing and the alarms would go off due to apnea of prematurity. I remember them needing caffeine to help them keep breathing. Every time an alarm went off, the nurse would come in and jiggle them or change their position and they would start breathing again. As I spent more and more time in the NICU, I started to recognize each alarm beep and what the nurses would do when the alarms went off. After a week or so, when an alarm went off, I would put my hand gently on their body and they would start to breathe again. It felt so empowering to help them.

Isaac continued growing and thriving except for having a low blood count. It was so painful to watch them draw blood from him every other day because I couldn't see any veins on him. I had to walk out of the room every time. Both of them needed NG tubes for feeding and actually that was our last milestone before we could take them home. Both of them were so tiny yet strong enough to pull out their NG tube multiple times.

I finally started changing diapers and holding them individually for kangaroo care. It felt good to be part of the team and contribute to their care.

It became a routine for us. We dropped off our 3-year-old son at preschool and I would go to the NICU. I would wait for rounds and then I would hold Eliza during her midmorning feeding. I would grab lunch and then I would hold Isaac in the afternoon. I was so excited to share the news with my husband's family that I was holding the babies. One of our family members told me to stay away from the babies because I was going to hurt them by holding them. That person told me I should let them stay in their incubator and let the doctors and nurses do their job. I stopped kangaroo care immediately.

Isaac's primary nurse noticed my hesitance to do kangaroo care and asked me what was going on. I shared my experience, and I was in tears and told her I was not trying to hurt my babies. She immediately paged the NICU doctor and shared my story. They assured me about all the benefits of kangaroo care and printed out some literature to share with my family members. I was so grateful for that because that was a cultural education we all shared in the NICU, and they supported me about educating family members.

One day, one of the nurses asked me if I wanted to hold both babies at the same time. She coordinated with both primary nurses the next day and collected all the necessary equipment in Isaac's room. As soon as I arrived, they all were happy to share that "today is the day you are going to hold both babies together." It was the best surprise ever. Isaac, Eliza, and I did so well, and we all felt calm and relaxed for the next 30 minutes just cuddling each other.

Spending almost 47 days in NICU made us a part of the NICU family. When you hear alarms going off in another baby's room or suddenly you see a baby getting wheeled away for emergency surgery, you drop on your knees and start praying for that baby and their family. It was no more my baby or their baby; we all have these miracle babies and they are fighters and we will pray for them all.

On day 47 we moved to the general pediatric floor because both babies were doing so well. Both twins had feeding issues; otherwise, they were meeting all their milestones. All they needed to do was take all their feedings by bottle for 24 hours and then they could go home.

The moment finally arrived. After 47 days in the NICU and over a week on the pediatric unit, we were going home with both babies—and without any tubes or equipment. We had multiple follow-up appointments to make sure both babies were thriving and growing appropriately.

I would not have survived without a great team in NICU. Nurses became my friends who reminded me that I hadn't eaten lunch that day and I needed self-care. Nurses were so kind and patient and encouraged us to become part of a care team and advocate for our babies. If my mom instinct was telling me something, they would bring my concerns to the doctors so it could be addressed. I did not receive the emotional support I needed from my family because they considered it my failure as a mom to be unable to keep the pregnancy until full term. My NICU nurses heard many of my stories and learned about the cultural expectations and challenges a mother like me faces when her babies are born prematurely. It was an educational experience for them because that side of maternal care was never verbalized. Now it has become part of their care plan to ask about cultural norms and differences.

Now Isaac and Eliza are 6½ years old and healthy thriving children. You cannot tell they were born at 27 weeks and 3 days. They participate in regular school activities and sports, and they are fun kids to be around. Eliza loves to write letters to her friends and family. Isaac loves to read books. They look up to their older brother. Their dad and I divorced in 2020 and all 3 kids managed this change well. You can tell NICU babies will thrive in any circumstances in their life. They are examples of never giving up and continuing to reach for their best.

Being a mom of NICU babies, I learned that every day is a blessing and a gift. Enjoy and make the most of it because no one knows what tomorrow will bring. Isaac and Eliza showed me that side of me, which I never knew I had in *me*. I finally understood the meaning of "God never gives you more than you can handle."

Parina, mother of Isaac and Eliza

Nathan

Born at 24 weeks, 4 days

Nathan on his birth day.

At 24 weeks 4 days' gestation, Nathan was born weighing just 1 pound 2 ounces. His premature birth was caused by ruptured membranes 15 weeks into the pregnancy. Miraculously, the pregnancy continued to viability, but due to his early birth, he was born with very immature lungs and the prognosis for long-term survival was grim.

Nathan had much to overcome. On his first day, he suffered from respiratory distress and a collapsed lung. At 1 week, Nathan suffered a bowel perforation, which ultimately resulted in him having surgery at 5 weeks old and just shy of 2 pounds. Almost as soon as he healed from the surgery, Nathan developed a severe form of retinopathy of prematurity and was given a 50% chance of going blind. Fortunately, he was able to receive treatment that successfully protected his vision and can see just as well as most other kids his age. Almost all of Nathan's major organ systems were affected by his prematurity. Nathan was lucky to have received excellent care during his NICU stay and I will be forever grateful to the wonderful doctors and nurses who cared for him when I couldn't.

Watching my son fight for his life in the hospital every day was incredibly hard, but the many magical moments I experienced with him as he got healthier and stronger kept me going. I will never forget the first time I held him in kangaroo care while he was still on a ventilator, the first time he took a full feed from a bottle with the breast milk I had pumped, and the first time I gave him a bath in a little bucket.

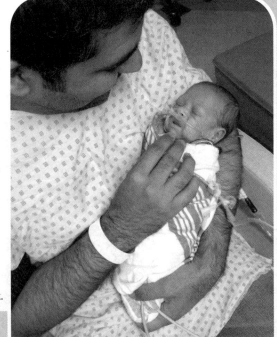

Nathan and his father have a talk.

After 140 days in the NICU, Nathan finally came home. It was a day of overwhelming happiness and gratitude but also one of fear that I was leaving behind the safety net of the NICU and would not know how to properly care for such a tiny being. Thankfully, the transition home went smoothly and I quickly learned how to manage the oxygen tank and apnea monitor that Nathan came home with and stayed on for a few months after leaving the NICU.

Nathan is an absolute joy in our family's life. Nathan has not only survived, but he's thriving. When he was

Nathan, at age 3.

only 2½ years old, Nathan began reading 3- and 4-letter words, and he's now learning to write, too. Nathan is loving, playful, and endlessly curious and has an infectious smile that can light up an entire room.

From the beginning, Nathan showed me his strength and resilience, which continues to inspire me every day. Having been blessed with the miracle of Nathan, my husband and I have established a nonprofit organization to provide support and resources to other families facing the challenges of preterm birth. Despite the harrowing ordeal we went through, we ended up with the greatest outcome we could have ever imagined—a handsome, sweet, and healthy little boy and the opportunity to help others in a meaningful way.

Cheryl and Sunil, parents of Nathan

Nathan and his parents.

Pascal

Born at 41 weeks, 2 days

Pascal was born by C-section and had Apgar scores of 8 and 9. In the recovery room, he was swaddled up in my arms when he turned blue-gray. They checked his oxygen, which seemed OK then. I remember in that moment feeling suspicious of him. I felt disconnected, looking at him from a distance. What was wrong with him? I thought we just had to get to being born, and then he would be OK.

When we moved to the postpartum room, he did it again. That time, his oxygen saturation was in the 60s. They took him to the nursery and then to the NICU. I could see him breathing really, really, really fast. I got to hold him skin-to-skin, with his nasal cannula and IV and monitor cables. When I had to go back to postpartum, I left him my T-shirt so he could still smell me. It felt incredibly wrong to be away from him. His labs strongly suggested infection, so his course of antibiotics was lengthened to 7 days. But that didn't mean we could go home after 7 days.

After a week, he had finished his course of antibiotics and weaned off his high-flow nasal cannula, and we started to work through the discharge process. I watched videos about CPR and safe sleep and set up his first pediatrician appointment. Pascal got set up for his car seat test. Even though he wasn't a preemie, because he'd had breathing problems,

Pascal snuggles with his dad's T-shirt in the NICU during phototherapy treatment.

he had to sit in the seat for 90 minutes without having oxygen desaturations. He failed miserably. Then he failed again. Then again. We ended up staying another 5 days while he got treatment for ongoing breathing problems. It was so hard to be so close to discharge and not be able to go home. You know those stages of grief? I kept going back and forth between acceptance and bargaining. "We don't live very far! I'll get a different stroller! I won't put him in a bouncy seat!" Each time he failed, his team would patiently explain that he wasn't safe to go home yet and that he just needed more time. Finally, on his fourth try, he kept his oxygen levels up, and that afternoon, after 11 days in the NICU, we went home!

Pascal is pretty healthy, though I still worry a lot when he gets sick, I think because it was so hard for him at the beginning. Our pediatrician understands where I'm coming from and helps me sort through my worry and reassures me about Pascal's health. He loves to climb, bang on boxes, and snuggle on my lap. It's hard to believe he needed so much help. I'm so grateful to the team who took care of him and can't wait to take him back to visit so they can see how much he's grown! **Read more about Pascal in "Where Are They Now?" in the Appendix.**

Alex, father of Pascal

CHAPTER 3

NICU Equipment and Tests

"As I spent more and more time in the NICU, I started to recognize each alarm beep and what the nurses would do when the alarms went off. After a week or so, when an alarm went off, I would put my hand gently on their bodies and they would start to breathe again. It felt so empowering to help them.

*Parina, mother of **Isaac** and **Eliza***

The equipment used for your baby's care in the neonatal intensive care unit (NICU) can be overwhelming for parents. Understanding the basics of NICU technology prepares you to ask questions about your baby's treatment and participate in care. The technology used in the NICU is important for your baby's survival, but it cannot replace the importance of your voice, your touch, and your involvement in your baby's plan of care.

Typical NICU Equipment

Just as the delivery area is set up with basic equipment for birth, the NICU is equipped with technology used to stabilize a baby's condition. Each baby's condition determines the type of support needed, but the following equipment and tests are commonly used.

Radiant Warmer and Incubator

The radiant warmer (left) and incubator (right) are designed to maintain the baby's temperature and enable the NICU team to easily observe and reach the baby. The radiant warmer has overhead heat and allows easy access to the baby from 3 sides. An incubator may have portholes to open, or the cover may lift off so you can touch your baby. An incubator maintains a constant warm temperature and humidified air. Most incubators and radiant warmers can also allow

thermostat control by measuring the baby's skin temperature through a small sensor taped to your baby's body. This temperature sensor is usually covered by a reflective adhesive material, often a circle of foil or a shiny gold heart. When your baby's skin has warmed to the preset temperature, the heat turns down; when your baby's skin temperature cools, the heat turns back up.

Radiant warmer.

Incubator.

> ❝ The first time I saw my daughter, I remember thinking how amazing it was that she looked like a completely healthy baby. She was just so tiny. Seeing the intubation tube and watching her chest rise and fall so rapidly was heart-wrenching. I just wanted to scoop her up and hold her close, but I couldn't. ❞
>
> *Kaitlynn, mother of **Sienna***

At 23 weeks' gestation, **Eliana** required intubation. Note the white cardiac monitor leads on her chest and the skin temperature sensor near her armpit. The white loops on her tummy are her umbilical catheters, inserted to deliver fluids and medication.

Cardiorespiratory Monitor and Electrocardiographic (ECG) Leads

Most babies in the NICU are placed on a *cardiorespiratory monitor* (sometimes called a *cardiac monitor* or, simply, a *monitor*). This device tracks the baby's vital signs, such as heart rate and breathing rate, and displays these numbers on a screen. This monitor will alert NICU staff to any variation. Three adhesive patches (*ECG leads*) are placed on the baby's chest and

One type of cardiorespiratory monitor.

abdomen or arms and legs (*limb leads*) and connected by cable to the monitor that displays the information on a screen. The monitor may also display oxygen saturation, if the baby has a pulse oximeter sensor attached, and blood pressure, if the baby has a blood pressure cuff or an *umbilical artery catheter* (*UAC*) in use.

Orogastric and Nasogastric Tubes

A thin, flexible tube inserted into your baby's mouth is called an *orogastric* (*OG*) tube. If it is inserted through the baby's nose, it is called a *nasogastric* (*NG*) tube. This tube goes down the food pipe (*esophagus*) and into the stomach. The tube may be used to release a buildup of gas and fluids from the baby's stomach (for example, during continuous positive airway pressure [CPAP]), or it may be used to deliver breast milk or formula to a baby who is not yet able to feed from the breast or bottle. When it is used for feeding, it may be called a *feeding tube* or *gavage tube*.

Ellie (left) and **Colson** (right) use their orogastric and nasogastric tubes (respectively) for feeding while they learn how to feed from the breast and bottle. When used for feeding, this tube is often called a *feeding tube* or *gavage tube*.

> One night I was changing Pascal's diaper, and he was flailing around, sticking his feet in the poop, grabbing at his IV, sneezing out his feeding tube, and it was one big giant mess. I think I ended up crying, pleading with him to leave the feeding tube alone, trying to slide it back in before it came out completely or got covered in poop. I could have called for a nurse. Maybe I should have done that, but I wanted so badly to be taking care of him.

*Alex, father of **Pascal***

Abel, born at 22 weeks and 5 days, also required intubation. Note the limb lead on each upper arm for cardiac monitoring and the shiny sticker that holds the skin temperature sensor in place.

Blood Pressure Cuff

Your baby's blood pressure may be taken in much the same way as your own. A small blood pressure cuff is wrapped around your baby's arm or leg, inflates, and measures the blood pressure. If your baby has a UAC, the blood pressure will be displayed on the cardiac monitor. (See Umbilical Artery Catheter [UAC] section for information about the UAC.)

Devices That Support Breathing and Oxygen Status

Many NICU babies require assistance with breathing. The devices described here provide different types of support depending on how much assistance the baby requires. Because of prematurity or illness, your newborn may need to breathe air with a higher concentration of oxygen than is available in "room air," which contains about 21% oxygen. Supplemental oxygen is any amount greater than 21% up to 100%. Supplemental oxygen, unless it is being used for a short period or set at a very low flow, is warmed and humidified. It can be given in several different ways.

Ventilator and Endotracheal Tube

A ventilator assists breathing for a baby who is having trouble breathing on their own. There are many types of ventilators, and each one works a little differently. The assisted breath is delivered through an *endotracheal (ET) tube* inserted into the baby's windpipe (*trachea*).

A ventilator can be adjusted to give the correct air–oxygen mixture, correct size of the breath (pressure, volume, and duration), and correct number of breaths per minute, depending on the baby's needs.

Eliana's endotracheal tube is secured by a device that holds the ET tube in her mouth and is taped to her cheeks. The ET tube is connected to long tubing that is connected to the ventilator nearby. The pulse oximeter cover is visible on her wrist.

Nasal Cannula

A *nasal cannula* is tubing that wraps around your baby's head and has prongs that fit into the baby's nose. A cannula can be used to deliver room air or supplemental oxygen in a variety of ways.

A cannula is a device used to deliver air, oxygen, CPAP, or noninvasive ventilation. On the left, **Alex** wears one style of nasal cannula. The prongs are clearly visible in his nose. On the right, **Eliana** wears a different style nasal cannula.

> " Take lots of pictures and videos and sneak a few of those tiny diapers to show people. They are blown away when they see the size of those diapers. "
>
> *Lisa, mother of **Frankie***

Continuous Positive Airway Pressure (CPAP)

A baby with CPAP breathes on their own, but CPAP keeps a steady stream of air pressure in the airway. This helps keep the tiny air sacs in the lungs from collapsing after each breath, making it easier for your baby to breathe. (See Chapter 5 for more information.) Most babies on CPAP also have an OG tube inserted through the mouth into the stomach. It is used to release the air that might get into the stomach and interfere with breathing.

Ellie (left), and **Eliana** (right) wear 2 different types of CPAP devices. Both have OG tubes to help release the air that might get into their stomachs.

Pulse Oximeter

Pulse oximetry may have been used in the delivery room if your baby needed resuscitation or supplemental oxygen. In the NICU, the pulse oximeter sensor wraps around your baby's hand, wrist, or foot. It uses a red light to measure the amount of oxygen attached to the hemoglobin molecules in your baby's blood. The measurement, called *oxygen saturation,* is displayed on the pulse oximeter screen along with your baby's heart rate. If your baby's oxygen saturation is outside the target range, the nurse or respiratory therapist may make an adjustment to the respiratory equipment.

The pulse oximeter shines a painless red light onto the baby's skin. The sensor is often covered with a soft cloth wrap to keep bright light in the room from interfering with the pulse oximeter signal.

Carbon Dioxide Transcutaneous Monitor

A *transcutaneous monitor* (*TCM*) may be used for monitoring carbon dioxide levels in the bloodstream. The TCM sensor lies on your baby's skin and warms the area under the sensor to "read" the amount of carbon dioxide in the blood. This can help determine if the baby needs additional help with breathing. Because of the warmth of the sensor, the TCM may leave a temporary red circle on your baby's skin.

The round plastic sensor and cable on the baby's forehead is a transcutaneous CO_2 monitor, used to monitor carbon dioxide levels in the blood.

Lines and Catheters

Because most babies in the NICU require fluids, medications, and nutrition via a blood vessel for some time after birth, they need some type of intravenous line or catheter. The type of device used depends on how long and for what purpose it is needed.

Intravenous Line

An *intravenous line* (often simply called an *IV*) is used to give your baby fluids, sugar, protein, salts and minerals (for example, sodium and potassium), and medications. Your

baby's IV may be placed in a vein in the hand or lower arm, foot or lower leg, or scalp. The IV can easily move out of place, allowing the IV fluid to leak into the tissue. This is called an *infiltrated IV*. If this happens, the IV must be taken out (*discontinued*) and restarted at another site. The nurse safeguards the IV so it functions at 1 site for as long as possible. Even under the best circumstances, an IV may last only a day or two.

An intravenous line is placed into a vein near the skin surface.

Umbilical Vein Catheter (UVC)

An *umbilical vein catheter* (*UVC*) is inserted into the umbilical vein, easily visible at the end of the umbilical cord, and advanced until it reaches a larger vein (the end of the *inferior vena*) just inside the baby's abdomen. An emergency UVC may be inserted if your baby needs to

have fluids or medications infused during resuscitation. A UVC may also be inserted if your baby needs an IV for more than a few days.

An umbilical catheter is a thin tube that can be threaded into an umbilical artery (umbilical artery catheter) or an umbilical vein (umbilical vein catheter). The umbilical catheter is often secured to the abdomen with a "bridge" of white tape. The shiny foil heart on the left holds the temperature sensor in place on the skin.

> ❝ Ellie's mouth was forced open by the plastic tubing down her throat, leads all over her chest, tape across her face and body, machines and tubes running in and out of her tiny plastic box. Ellie looked like an experiment out of a sci-fi movie, and it was almost too overwhelming for me. ❞
>
> *Melissa, mother of **Ellie***

Peripherally Inserted Central Catheter (PICC line)

A *peripherally inserted central catheter* (*PICC* [pick]) *line*, or *central line*, is used when your baby needs an IV for longer than a few days. It is inserted into the arm or leg and threaded into a larger blood vessel deep inside the body. The PICC line is used to give medicines, fluids, and nutrients over a longer period, usually a week or more.

The peripherally inserted central catheter (PICC line) is the thin white tubing on this baby's left leg. This baby also has a pulse oximeter sensor and sensor cover on her right foot.

> ❝ One of my regrets was declining the PICC line when it was offered. A PICC line seemed invasive and scary, but that IV was really hard to keep in. How does a newborn have enough coordination to gnaw on his own IV? He was a big chunky baby and IV placements were frequent and difficult. ❞
>
> *Alex, father of **Pascal***

Arterial Line

If the NICU team needs continuous monitoring of your baby's blood pressure, they may place an *arterial line*. An arterial line is a special catheter that is threaded into an artery and then attached to an electronic monitor. In the NICU, arterial lines are frequently placed into an artery in the wrist or ankle.

Umbilical Artery Catheter (UAC)

A UAC is inserted into 1 of the 2 arteries that are easily visible at the end of the umbilical cord and advanced until it reaches a large artery (the *aorta*). A UAC is placed if your baby requires frequent blood testing or continuous blood pressure measurement.

Basic NICU Tests

The NICU team uses many different tests to get information about your baby's health.

Imaging Tests

X-rays

X-rays (also called radiographs) are an important diagnostic tool in the NICU. X-rays are used to confirm the correct position of tubes and catheters, such as the endotracheal tube and umbilical catheter, if one is in place. X-rays also allow care providers to assess the condition of the lungs and some abdominal organs.

Although your baby is exposed to a certain amount of radiation with every x-ray , the amount is carefully controlled in relation to your baby's size and weight. Unnecessary x-rays are avoided. If the baby's genital area is in the primary x-ray beam, it is shielded with a lead cover.

Ultrasound

Just like ultrasound tests used during pregnancy, *ultrasonography* may be used to look at various organs, including your baby's brain, heart, lungs, liver, intestines, and kidneys. Sometimes, the ultrasound machine will be used to help guide the medical team as they perform procedures. The ultrasound machine uses sound waves instead of radiation.

Blood Tests

Blood Culture

If the team suspects your baby may have an infection, a sample of blood will be taken and sent for a *blood culture*. The blood sample is placed in a bottle and sent to the laboratory, where it is watched for several days for signs of bacterial (or fungal) growth. Bacteria often take 1 to 3 days to grow, and a fungus may take longer (a week or more). If there is no sign of bacterial growth, the culture is called *negative*. In this case, negative is a good thing. Viruses are different from bacteria and require special kinds of culture methods. At times, your team may obtain blood or other samples for viral culture.

Blood Gas

A *blood gas* is a test that uses a small amount of blood to check the levels of oxygen, carbon dioxide, and acid. The blood can be sampled from different sources: artery, vein, or capillary. An *arterial blood gas* (*ABG*) requires health care professionals to use a syringe and needle to obtain blood from an artery. Other times, a *venous blood gas* (*VBG*) may be obtained from a vein using a syringe and a needle. A cap gas (short for *capillary blood gas* or *CBG*), which is obtained by pricking your baby's heel with a small puncture device, may be sufficient. If blood gas levels are needed frequently, the team may insert a UAC or UVC and obtain the sample through the catheter, avoiding the need to puncture your baby's skin for each sample.

Blood gas results are commonly used to help the team check your baby's lung function and adjust the ventilator settings. A blood gas test can also give the team valuable information about your baby's metabolism, hydration, and nutrition.

Complete Blood Cell Count

A *complete blood cell count* (*CBC*) is a test to measure the different components of your baby's blood, including the amount of red blood cells (*hematocrit* and *hemoglobin*), white blood cells, and platelets. Red blood cells carry oxygen to tissues. When they are low, it means the baby has *anemia*. White blood cells fight infection. If they are very low or very high, it may be a sign of infection. Platelets are part of the system that makes blood clot and controls bleeding.

Electrolytes

Electrolytes (sometimes called *lytes*) measure the balance of salts and minerals in your baby's blood. Measuring electrolytes helps the team adjust the fluids and nutrition your baby receives and assess how well the kidneys are functioning.

Glucose (Blood Sugar)

A *blood glucose* test measures the amount of sugar in your baby's blood. Frequently, the test is done at the bedside using a small drop of blood from your baby's heel. If the number is unusually high or low, a sample may be obtained from a blood vessel and sent to the laboratory for more precise analysis.

Newborn Metabolic Screening (State Screening)

All newborns in the United States have a blood sample obtained shortly after birth. The blood is placed onto a special piece of paper. The sample is sent to a central laboratory, usually in the same state, and tested for a wide range of inherited diseases. Many of these tests are looking for rare but important abnormalities of hormones and metabolism. It is common for babies in the NICU to have temporary abnormalities on these tests called *false positives*. If a component of the metabolic screen is abnormal, someone from the laboratory may contact you and your baby's doctor by phone. Your doctor will explain the test result and the follow-up plan.

Sepsis Evaluation

Right after birth, or later if your baby's condition changes, the care team may need to determine if your baby has an infection. Looking for laboratory signs of infection is often called a *sepsis evaluation*. The team will order a variety of blood tests (as described previously) and possibly obtain urine and spinal fluid samples.

Spinal Fluid

If the team suspects your baby may have an infection, they may also want to obtain a sample of *cerebrospinal fluid* (CSF). CSF is the clear fluid that surrounds your brain and spinal cord. If this fluid is infected, it is called *meningitis*. The sample is obtained by inserting a very small needle into the baby's back between the vertebrae. This procedure is called a *lumbar puncture* (LP).

Urine Tests

Kidneys are very sensitive to changes in the body. The amount of urine and what is in it can tell the NICU team much about your baby's general condition and progress after birth. If a urine sample is needed, a specially designed plastic bag may be taped over your baby's labia or penis and scrotum. When the baby urinates, the urine collects in the bag and is sent to the laboratory for analysis. This type of urine collection is called a *clean catch* and is used to check the urine for sugar, salts, or blood.

If infection is a concern, a urine culture may be done. The urine sample may be collected by inserting a small sterile catheter into the baby's bladder through the opening where urine comes out (the baby's *urethra*) and withdrawing the urine. Sometimes, it is very difficult to insert a sterile catheter into a small baby's urethra. In this case, another method is used that involves inserting a needle through the baby's lower abdomen and directly into the bladder. This technique is called a *suprapubic* or *bladder tap*.

> Ironically, I had planned for an intervention-free birth before Auggie's early arrival. Because of his early arrival, I am forever grateful for the medical technology and clinical expertise we were afforded and for all of the care he received in the NICU from such dedicated and compassionate nurses and other staff.
>
> *Robyn, mother of **Auggie***

The Importance of Parenting

The NICU you enter today is very different from the NICU of even a few years ago. Advances in respiratory care, monitoring, and diagnostic techniques have been incredible. This technology can be overwhelming for parents, but the NICU team will answer your questions, help you get acquainted with your baby despite the wires and cables, and guide you as you learn about equipment and procedures. Soon, you'll know the purpose of each device and what each sound means. Paying attention to your baby is more important than watching the monitors!

Meridith

Born at 31 weeks, 5 days

Our journey to becoming parents began with a positive pregnancy test less than a year after a devastating miscarriage. The pregnancy was, for the most part, uneventful up until our 20-week ultrasound. My husband Joe and I opted not to find out the gender, so it was strictly an anatomy scan. Our ultrasound was normal other than having a hard time finding her kidneys. We would find out after her birth that the reason they couldn't find them was they were hypoplastic, meaning small for her age.

All was well until I was 31 weeks and 3 days pregnant, which was a Friday. I was at work, having back pain and was a little uncomfortable, but I boiled it down to being 31 weeks pregnant. I left work to have dinner out and to do some shopping with Joe, but I was still feeling a little uncomfortable. We decided to forgo shopping and go home.

I tried a hot shower and lying down, but nothing seemed to help. After trying to get some rest, we decided it was time to call triage. They told me to come and get checked out, just in case. When I arrived in triage, it was confirmed that I was in preterm labor.

I was admitted and received my first dose of betamethasone Saturday morning, as well as something to help stop my labor. At this point, we were concerned for our baby but knew we were in the right hands. Later that evening everyone on my team was confident that they had successfully stopped my contractions. There was even talk of sending me home on Sunday to continue bedrest for the rest of my pregnancy.

Meridith had other plans. Shortly after 5 am on Sunday, I felt a lot of pressure and was having contractions again. My nurse checked me, and I was almost completely dilated. The decision was made to move me to the OR, to be close to the NEST (Newborn Evaluation, Stabilization, and Treatment) area when she was born. After a short period of pushing, Meridith was born at 31 weeks, 5 days and weighed 4 pounds 3 ounces. She wasn't crying initially, so I wasn't able to see her before they took her to the NEST. After confirming that I was okay, Joe followed her out to the NEST while they finished with me in the OR.

After what seemed like forever, I was wheeled out of the OR and into the NEST to see and hold my sweet girl and have our first family picture. At that moment, I knew our journey

Meridith on CPAP at 1 day of age.

Meridith, 8 months old, develops her musical talent.

to take her home would take a little longer than expected, but we had an excellent care team and wonderful support, so we knew she would make it home. I was eventually taken back to my room to recover.

Later that day, we made our way to the NICU to see Meridith. Seeing her snuggled in her closed incubator, with her continuous positive airway pressure (CPAP) mask on and all her tubes and wires made me sad. Why did my body fail to keep her safe inside me until she was due? We were asked if we wanted to hold her and our answer was a resounding yes! We both had an opportunity to do skin-to-skin with her, which was the best feeling. It was the first time Joe had gotten to hold her, and seeing him hold her was so heartwarming. She already had Daddy wrapped around her little finger.

Thankfully, she didn't have to be on CPAP for very long, and then she went to a nasal cannula. It was a little easier to manage and I can only imagine more comfortable for her as well. However, that day her bilirubin was high enough that she had to go under phototherapy, which unfortunately limited the amount of time we got to hold her.

Four days after she was born, we met with a nephrologist (kidney specialist). Due to her creatinine level being high and continuing to climb, it had been determined that her kidneys were small for her size. At that time, the nephrologist was hopeful that her kidneys were just slow to wake up from her premature birth, but, as time passed, it became clear that was not the case. Thus began our journey with chronic kidney disease (CKD), which made the next part of our journey more complicated.

On day 5, I was finally able to attempt breastfeeding, something I had been looking forward to since I found out I was pregnant. The first attempt showed a lot of promise; she latched well, despite the prematurity, feeding tube in her mouth, and nasal cannula. I was crying I was so happy. That, unfortunately, would be one of the last times she nursed well, which took a huge emotional toll.

To treat her CKD, they increased her fluid intake and calories, which meant she was never hungry, so despite our best efforts and a lot of help from her care team, Meridith just wasn't interested in breastfeeding. Even though I couldn't feed her directly, I was able to pump for almost 3 years. Drinking her bottles of fortified breast milk was a struggle as well, so a good percentage was fed through an NG tube in her nose.

After the first week, my husband returned to work to save his time for when we were discharged but he would come and visit us before and after work, then go home to take care of the pets and house.

Our next big scare came on day 11 of our NICU stay. Meridith's lab work was off, she was requiring more oxygen than normal and was rather sleepy, which prompted a septic work-up. I had to wait outside the room by myself since my husband was at work. Thankfully, my sister-in-law happened to visit on one of her breaks, so I had her for support. During the spinal tap, I couldn't see Meridith, but I could hear her crying like I'd never heard her cry before, and it was heart wrenching not being able to comfort her. I couldn't wait to get back in there to snuggle her. Thankfully, it turned out she didn't have sepsis but while we waited for the results, she had to be put on high-strength antibiotics, which weren't good for her kidney function. That was a bit stressful knowing that the longer she was on them, the more damage that could be done to her already compromised kidneys.

After that day, her NICU stay was routine. She was learning to suck, swallow, and breathe. She was on and off the nasal cannula a few times and it was determined that she still needed the extra support, which was likely from her preemie lungs and the extra fluid needed to support her kidneys.

The first week in February, we started to talk about going home. She just needed to eat a little bit more per feed and trial again off her oxygen, as well as do the routine discharge items, such as her car seat test, hearing test, our CPR class, and so forth. Finally, February 6 came around and she still kind of stalled on everything, so our team asked if we would be okay taking her home on ¼ liter of oxygen and an NG tube for her feeds. My husband and I talked it over and were over the moon happy to take her home so we could be together as a family, albeit a little nervous about the oxygen and NG tube.

Before we could discharge home with an NG tube, Joe and I had to demonstrate that we could put another one in, for routine changes and when Meridith accidentally pulled out her tube (which, it turns out, happened a lot; we got to be very good at it). We both were able to do it and the next day was going-home day! After 34 days in the NICU, we had finally reached the day we had been looking forward to for a long time. Throughout our stay in the NICU, the nurses, doctors, and other staff had become like family to us, so it was somewhat bittersweet.

Those first few days at home were spent adjusting to having a newborn with oxygen and a feeding tube. The first few nights were a little rough worrying about her being off the monitors. Thankfully though, everything went smoothly.

Two years after her NICU discharge, it became clear that her fluid intake was going to be too much for her to be able to drink on her own, so we opted to have her NG tube switched to a g-tube. We wished we had done it sooner, as it was so much easier to manage and the risk of her pulling it out was much lower. With the change to the G-tube, we were able to switch her from just the breastmilk fortified with formula to a breastmilk and blended diet that consisted of real food. She blossomed on her new diet.

Our years since discharge have included many visits to her pediatrician, nephrologist, pulmonologist, and, most recently, her endocrinologist. Meridith is a smart, loving, resilient, strong young lady who is thriving!

Mary Ellen and Joe, parents of Meridith

Meridith at age 7 (in front of her dad), with her sister Clara and her mother.

August

(Auggie)

Born at 24 weeks

Auggie was born at 24 weeks of gestation. He weighed 1 pound 13 ounces at birth and spent his first 131 days of life in the Infant Special Care Unit.

Just before the 24-week mark, I started experiencing some very faint discharge. At first I thought I was overreacting and that it was likely a normal reaction of my body to a pregnancy at that stage. Thankfully, I listened to that little voice in the back of my head and called my midwife. It was in that moment that everything related to our birth plan unraveled, every vision or plan for a healthy, uncomplicated birth experience vanished. I was admitted to the hospital and soon after, I had a placental abruption and an emergency C-section.

Robyn holds Auggie for the first time.

Auggie was handed off to the neonatology team for resuscitation and they worked quickly to save him. I don't think we fully understood until much later just how important those first few minutes were in determining whether he would survive.

We would not hold our son for 2 weeks and spent the next 4½ months making daily visits to the NICU to see him, multiple calls per day to get updates on his progress, and taking it all one day at a time. It was the longest 131 days of our life.

The way we became parents to Auggie was hard; it was emotionally exhausting, and that lasted well after the physical pain from the aftermath of his birth. It's hard on marriages to start your life-changing journey as parents while your baby is still in the NICU. I had a lot of guilt and lingering emotional stress and didn't quite know how to process it all. My husband processed his emotions differently, so it was a strain and it was frustrating to both of us to understand one another's vastly different expressions. I felt guilty, as though it were somehow my fault that my baby was born in such a fragile state, with his life in the balance. I was hard on myself.

One thing I wish I knew earlier on during our journey was to ask for help and to accept that post-traumatic stress disorder (PTSD) is very much something that NICU parents can experience. There were horrible flashbacks and guttural cries, initially, thinking about the horrible nightmare of his birth and the short time leading up to his birth. We didn't know

Auggie spent 4½ months in the NICU.

if he would live or if his quality of life would be "good" if he did live. I still find it difficult to relate to women who have uncomplicated, full-term births. I didn't experience a third trimester of pregnancy.

Another thing I have forgiven myself for, but didn't at the time, was my inability to love my son in the first few weeks. At 24 weeks' gestation, he didn't look like the babies you see in pictures or on social media. It was a defense mechanism, I think. I didn't have anyone in my social network who had had a baby so early, or even preterm at all. That was isolating. There was so much anticipation and buildup for our son's discharge from the NICU that by the time the day arrived, I was surprised by my sudden sadness to leave the place I so desperately wanted to flee. I was sad to leave the nurses, who we could never thank enough for their care of our child. Bringing Auggie home had its own challenges, however; we worried constantly those first few months about his development, whether he was getting the right nutrition, and whether he'd contract some illness.

Years later, I still marvel at his auspicious beginnings in life and how remarkably he's overcome all of the hurdles in his way. We will admit that we have one of the best-case outcomes; Auggie does not have any lingering physical or mental developmental delays. I'm always cognizant of the fact that there are many NICU families dealing with more severe complications of their children's early births. That's never lost on me. I'd do it all over again because I have this amazing, smart, funny, curious, friendly, compassionate little person who is our son. I'm in awe of him, that we get to be his. He's like the best gift that I never quite feel I deserve. **Read more about August (Auggie) in "Where Are They Now?" in the Appendix.**

Robyn, mother of Auggie

Auggie, at age 2½ years.

CHAPTER 4

Common Medical Problems

> Logan was only 6 weeks early,
> which was nothing compared to some of
> the very premature babies in the NICU.
> Still, so many thoughts were running
> through my head: What if I hurt him?
> Would he be okay? Why did he need all
> this equipment? Was I not a good mother
> housing him for only 34 weeks?
> What did I do wrong?
>
> *Christina, mother of **Logan***

This chapter will help explain some of the medical problems that babies will have in the NICU. Preterm and full-term newborns can have these problems. Some of the problems that are specific to preterm babies are discussed in the next chapter.

Some babies will never have any of the problems discussed in this chapter, while others may face many challenges. The descriptions in this chapter are brief and include some of the most common findings and treatments for each problem. Each baby is different, and your baby's situation may differ a little or a lot from the descriptions you read here. Your NICU team can provide you with more specific details about your baby.

Problems With Breathing

Transient Tachypnea of the Newborn (TTN)

During development, the fetal lungs are filled with fluid, not air. During the process of labor and birth, most of this fluid is removed. *Transient tachypnea of the newborn (TTN)*, or *wet lung*, develops when fluid remains in the newborn's lungs after birth. Babies born by cesarean or rapid vaginal delivery are at increased risk for developing TTN.

Potential Problems Caused by TTN

Fluid in the lungs may cause your baby to breathe fast. Fast breathing is called *tachypnea*. It may also make breathing more difficult causing the skin and muscles on your baby's chest to suck inward between the ribs with each breath. Labored breathing may also cause babies to make grunting sounds when breathing.

The additional work of breathing is tiring and makes it hard to get enough oxygen and get rid of carbon dioxide. Rapid breathing also makes sucking and swallowing difficult and may make it very hard for your baby to eat.

Diagnosis and Treatment of TTN

A chest x-ray (*radiograph*) may look hazy and show signs of fluid in the lungs. To help with breathing, some babies with TTN require additional oxygen or a small amount of continuous positive airway pressure (CPAP) given through a mask or small prongs in the baby's nose. Transient tachypnea of the newborn and pneumonia can appear very similar on a chest x-ray, so your baby may receive antibiotics if the medical team considers pneumonia a possibility. Babies with TTN may need intravenous (IV) fluids until their breathing slows down. Usually, TTN resolves within a couple of days and does not lead to any lasting problems.

Meconium Aspiration Syndrome (MAS)

Meconium is a sterile, dark-green, sticky substance produced in the fetal bowel and passed in the baby's first few stools (bowel movements) after birth. Sometimes, the baby passes meconium while still in the uterus. In other words, the baby poops for the first time in the uterus. The poop makes the amniotic fluid, which is usually clear, a greenish-brown color. This is called *meconium-stained amniotic fluid* (*MSAF*).

Meconium-stained amniotic fluid is more common when the pregnancy goes late (*post-term*) and may be a sign of fetal distress. After the fetus passes meconium, MSAF may get into the mouth and airway before or right after birth. Babies who get a large amount of meconium into their lungs can have severe breathing problems after birth. This condition is called *meconium aspiration syndrome* (*MAS*). About 10% of all babies pass meconium in the amniotic fluid, but only a small number have breathing problems.

Resuscitation of Babies With Meconium-Stained Amniotic Fluid

Until recently, if a baby with MSAF was born limp and not breathing, a tube was inserted into the windpipe (*endotracheal intubation*) and suction was applied to remove meconium from the airway. Research has *not* shown that *intubation* and *tracheal suction* prevent MAS, and routinely inserting a tube into the windpipe with the aim of removing meconium is no longer recommended.

Symptoms of MAS

After birth, the meconium-stained amniotic fluid may temporarily stain the baby's skin, fingernails, or umbilical cord a greenish color. Babies who have inhaled meconium into their lungs may need help to breathe after birth. They may have rapid breathing (*tachypnea*), blue color of the body and around the mouth (*cyanosis*), widely opened nostrils with each breath (*nasal flaring*), and increased work of breathing resulting in the drawing in of the chest wall with each breath (*retractions*).

Potential Complications of MAS

The complications of meconium aspiration will depend on the baby's degree of distress before birth and the severity of MAS.

Mild meconium aspiration usually resolves with few problems. Babies with mild meconium aspiration may need extra oxygen and IV fluids for several hours to days following birth. If your baby is breathing rapidly, feeding may be delayed and IV fluid may be necessary.

More severe cases of MAS can make a baby very sick. Meconium is irritating to the lungs, and although it is sterile, it may encourage an infection. Some babies may develop a problem called *persistent pulmonary hypertension of the newborn* (*PPHN*), described later in this chapter.

Babies with severe MAS may need a breathing tube inserted in their windpipe (*endotracheal intubation*), a ventilator to assist breathing, antibiotics, and treatments to relax the blood vessels in their lungs. Giving *surfactant* into the lungs may help improve lung function (see Chapter 5). Sometimes, babies are given oxygen mixed with a gas called *nitric oxide* to help relax the blood vessels in the lungs (see the Treatment for PPHN section for more information about nitric oxide). Meconium may trap air in the tiny breathing sacs of the lung (*alveoli*), causing them to rupture and leak air into the spaces around the lung. Babies with the most severe MAS may need to be transferred to a higher-level, specialized NICU for a temporary form of heart–lung bypass called *extracorporeal membrane oxygenation* (*ECMO*) (explained later in this chapter).

Air Leaks

When a baby has trouble breathing, one possible complication is an *air leak*. This occurs when air ruptures 1 or more of the breathing sacs of the lung *(alveoli)* and air leaks into the spaces around the lung tissue. Air that collects between the lung and rib cage is called a *pneumothorax* and may cause the lung to collapse.

Babies at Risk for Air Leaks

Some healthy babies will develop an air leak when they inflate their lungs with their first breaths after birth. Others will develop an air leak because they have excess fluid or meconium in their lungs. Babies who need breathing support from CPAP or a ventilator are at a higher risk of developing an air leak because of the mechanical pressure within their lungs. Preterm babies are also at higher risk because their lungs are stiffer at birth.

Signs of an Air Leak

Some babies with an air leak have no signs or only mild rapid breathing (*tachypnea*). Other babies show more signs of distress, including low heart rate (*bradycardia*), labored breathing, low blood pressure (*hypotension*), and decreased oxygen saturation.

Diagnosis of Air Leaks

A chest x-ray is used to diagnose air leaks. If a baby suddenly has respiratory distress, a bright light may be shined on the chest to look for a "glow" that indicates a collection of air outside the lung. This procedure is called *transillumination*. Although the result is not as specific as a chest x-ray, transillumination can usually be done more quickly in an emergency.

Treatment for Air Leaks

Newborns with a small air leak and no significant breathing problems do not require any treatment. If the air leak causes more significant breathing problems, the air can be removed by inserting a needle into the chest and pulling out the air with a syringe. This procedure is called *needle aspiration* or *needle thoracentesis*. If there is concern that the air may keep leaking, a thin plastic or silicone tube (*chest tube*) attached to a suction device can be left in the chest to remove the leaking air. In most cases, the damaged alveoli repair themselves within several days and the chest tube can be removed.

The white tube coming from the baby's chest is a chest tube and is used to treat a pneumothorax. This baby also has a transcutaneous CO_2 monitor on their forehead, an endotracheal tube secured to their face, and an umbilical catheter secured with white tape just above the diaper.

Persistent Pulmonary Hypertension of the Newborn (PPHN)

Before birth, the fetus does not use their lungs, and the blood vessels leading to the lungs are tightly squeezed (*constricted*). After birth, babies take their first breaths and fill their lungs with air, and the blood vessels normally relax. *Persistent pulmonary hypertension of the newborn (PPHN)* occurs when the blood vessels do not relax and blood cannot get into the lungs. This decreases the oxygen supply to the newborn's body and can be a life-threatening problem.

Babies who have trouble breathing after birth are at risk of developing PPHN. The signs of PPHN look a lot like signs of other major illnesses. In addition to difficulty breathing, your baby may have low blood pressure or look pale, blue, or blotchy (*mottled*).

Diagnosis of PPHN

If your baby requires very high amounts of additional oxygen to maintain normal blood oxygen levels, PPHN may be suspected. A cardiac ultrasound (*echocardiogram*) is often done to look at how well the heart is working. The echocardiogram looks at how well the blood is flowing to the lungs and estimates the pressure in the heart and major blood vessels.

Treatment for PPHN

The goals of treatment are to relax the blood vessels in the lungs and improve oxygen levels in the blood. Babies often need help from a ventilator, and there are many types. The medical team may use a special ventilator called a *high-frequency* ventilator that provides very rapid breaths with vibrations or small puffs of air. Medications may be needed to improve the baby's heart function, raise the baby's blood pressure, or help the baby sleep and relieve any discomfort.

Other possible treatments for severe PPHN include the use of *inhaled nitric oxide* or *ECMO*.

Nitric Oxide (NO)

Nitric oxide is an important chemical in the body that helps regulate blood pressure. When breathed into the lungs, nitric oxide relaxes the blood vessels in the lungs and can improve oxygen entry. Note that nitric oxide sounds similar but is *not* the same as nitrous oxide or "laughing gas."

Extracorporeal Membrane Oxygenation (ECMO)

Extracorporeal membrane oxygenation (*ECMO* [EK-mo]) is considered for babies if other treatments have not been successful. ECMO is a type of temporary heart–lung bypass that allows the baby's lungs (and sometimes the heart) to rest so they can recover. The machine used for ECMO is similar to the machine used for open-heart surgery and requires 1 or 2 large tubes (*cannulas*) to be surgically placed in large blood vessels in the baby's neck. Extracorporeal membrane oxygenation is surgically and technically complex and is not available at every NICU; therefore, if ECMO therapy is required, your baby may be transferred to a higher-level, specialized NICU.

Ellie is on ECMO. She has had 2 tubes (cannulas) surgically placed into large blood vessels in her neck (visible on the lower left). Her support includes an endotracheal tube, umbilical catheters, and numerous intravenous lines.

> How was this the same perfect baby I had just delivered 2 hours ago, whose blue eyes had opened so perfectly and looked into mine? I placed my hand on her and tried to imagine she was just like my other 2 children but couldn't get past the situation in front of me. My heart was breaking.

Melissa, mother of **Ellie**

When an infant is on ECMO, the lungs are no longer the main way that the baby breathes, although the newborn may still remain intubated and receive some breathing support from

a ventilator at low settings. Babies need to remain quiet and may receive pain medications, as well as sedatives, to ensure comfort. How long a newborn remains on ECMO varies depending on the clinical condition and recovery of heart and lung function. Most newborns are on ECMO for 5 to 7 days, but some will need ECMO for much longer.

Although ECMO can be lifesaving, there are risks associated with it. These include bleeding, forming of blood clots, and kidney failure. The blood vessel used for ECMO cannulas may be permanently blocked after ECMO, and this can pose a risk for future problems.

The typical amount of equipment at the bedside of a newborn on ECMO.

Problems With Infections

Our immune system protects us from infection. The body has many defense mechanisms to prevent things like bacteria and viruses from invading. Because the defense mechanisms of babies are still immature, newborns are at greater risk of developing an infection than are older children or adults.

Why Babies Are at Risk

The skin and mucous membranes that line the respiratory system and gut help to keep potential invaders out. If foreign bodies get past these barriers, white blood cells, antibodies, and other substances in the blood are called into action to find and attack them.

Some risk factors for infection can be identified before the baby is born. If there are signs of infection in the amniotic fluid during labor or the baby is born preterm, the risk of early newborn infection is significantly increased. Preterm newborns are at a greater risk of developing infections during their first weeks after birth because all of their defense mechanisms are immature. Their skin does not form a complete barrier, their white blood cells are not as effective at killing invaders, and they have fewer antibodies in their blood. Antibodies are transferred across the placenta to the fetus during the third trimester of pregnancy, but many preterm babies are born before this happens.

Babies in the NICU, in general, are at risk for infection during their hospital stay. Some of the medical equipment and procedures that babies in the NICU need to survive, including breathing tubes, feeding tubes, and IV lines, interfere with their protective barriers and increase the risk of infection.

Risk Factors for Early Newborn Infection

- Prematurity
- Preterm or prolonged rupture of amniotic membranes
- Maternal fever
- Infection of the placenta and amniotic fluid (*chorioamnionitis*)
- Maternal colonization with group B β-hemolytic streptococcus (*group B strep*)
- Previous baby with infection in the newborn period

Signs of Possible Infection in the Newborn

- Difficulty breathing
- Breathing pauses (apnea)
- Limp muscle tone (hypotonia)
- Lack of energy (lethargy)
- Irritability or fussiness
- Seizures
- Vomiting
- Pale, mottled, or blotchy skin
- Low body temperature
- Fever
- Low blood pressure (hypotension)
- Low blood sugar (hypoglycemia)
- High blood sugar (hyperglycemia)
- Rapidly appearing yellow skin (jaundice)

> ❝ I figured out that in order to survive such an unpredictable NICU journey, it would be best to have no expectations. The ups and downs are like a roller coaster, and the lows are very low. I learned that every day is a blessing, no matter what it brings. ❞
>
> *Shana, mother of* **Abel**

Signs of Infection

Babies with an infection often show general signs of illness or signs that mimic other problems. These may be subtle or quite dramatic, depending on the severity and type of infection. Some signs of infection can be difficult to separate from normal preterm baby behaviors.

Diagnosis of Infection

If the NICU team suspects your baby has a bacterial infection, they will do a *sepsis evaluation* (also called *sepsis work-up*). They take samples of your baby's body fluids and send them to the laboratory to see if bacteria can be identified. Depending on your baby's age and signs of infection, they may take samples of blood, urine, and spinal fluid for culture testing.

The laboratory monitors the cultures and will contact the NICU team if there are signs of bacterial growth. It commonly takes 12 to 48 hours in the laboratory before a culture shows any signs of bacterial growth. If nothing grows, the culture is *negative*.

Other blood tests, such as a blood cell count, and x-ray of the chest or belly may also be done. At times, the team may be concerned about less common types of infections, including very slow growing bacteria, viruses, and fungi (yeast). If the team suspects one of these infections, they may send additional samples for cultures and other tests.

> ❝ Holland took a turn for the worse when she was about a week old. Her platelet count dropped rather suddenly, and the doctors suspected she had an infection. The next 2 days were really long, stressful days, and we did not get a lot of good news. It was very disheartening. Finally, on day 4, Holland's platelet count improved! Through it all, Holland was a really tough cookie. All of her tiny little parts continued to function and she plugged right along. ❞
>
> *Billie, mother of* **Holland** *and* **Eden**

Treatment for Infection

The treatment for bacterial infection is antibiotics—medications that are effective against bacteria. First, your baby receives antibiotics that are effective against many different types of bacteria (*broad-spectrum antibiotics*). As the medical team learns more about the type of bacteria causing your baby's infection, they may give a more specific antibiotic. If your baby needs treatment for a virus or fungus, other medications will be added to the treatment plan.

Supportive care is also provided to increase your baby's ability to fight the infection. A warm environment, IV fluids, medicines to maintain normal blood pressure, adequate nutrition (oral or IV), and oxygen or assisted breathing are examples of supportive care.

Two Specific Infections: Group B β-Hemolytic Streptococcus and Central Line–Associated Bloodstream Infection

Group B β-Hemolytic Streptococcus

Group B β-hemolytic streptococcus (*GBS*; also called *group B strep*) is a type of bacteria found in the birth canal or rectum in about 10% to 30% of healthy women. This organism usually does not cause any symptoms or illness in the pregnant person but, in some cases, may be responsible for urinary tract infection or infection of the amniotic membranes that surround the baby before birth (*chorioamnionitis*).

Pregnant people are screened for GBS at about 35 to 37 weeks of pregnancy. If a pregnant person carries this organism in their vagina or rectum, antibiotics are given during labor to help prevent the spread of GBS to the baby. Without antibiotics, some babies born to pregnant people with GBS bacteria will develop a serious infection. The overall risk is about 1 in 100 babies, but the risk to an individual baby is much lower or much higher than that, depending on how long before birth the water is broken (*membranes ruptured)* and whether or not a fever develops during labor. The risk is even higher if the baby is born preterm, if there is a large number of GBS bacteria present in the vagina or rectum, if a urinary tract infection with GBS was diagnosed during the pregnancy, or if a previous baby had a GBS infection. When antibiotics are given during labor, the risk of the baby becoming infected is decreased almost 100-fold. If a planned cesarean delivery is performed before labor starts and before membranes are ruptured, the risk of GBS infection is very low and antibiotics are not given.

Group B strep infection in the newborn can cause blood infection, pneumonia, a severe whole-body reaction to infection (*sepsis*), or infection of the spinal fluid (*meningitis*). Even though only a small number of babies exposed to GBS develop an infection, those who become infected can be seriously ill, with rapid progression to severe breathing difficulty and shock.

There are 2 periods after birth when GBS infections typically occur: *early-onset* refers to the first week after birth, and *late-onset* GBS typically occurs at 3 to 4 weeks of age, although late-onset GBS infection can occur anytime between 7 days and 3 months of age. Early-onset GBS is best prevented by giving antibiotics during labor to pregnant people who have a positive GBS screening test result. Late-onset GBS infection cannot be prevented but may be suspected when a baby shows signs of infection.

Central Line–Associated Bloodstream Infection

Central line–associated bloodstream infection (*CLABSI* [KLAB-see]) is a term used to describe a bacterial infection in the bloodstream of a baby who has a catheter placed in a major blood vessel (*central line*). These lines are frequently used in the NICU and include umbilical catheters and peripherally inserted central catheters (PICC lines).

The most common bacteria causing CLABSI are *staphylococci*, which normally live on the baby's skin. Most babies with CLABSI do not develop sudden or extreme signs of infection. Instead, they may gradually have more episodes of apnea or feeding problems. Sometimes, parents and the medical team say that the baby "just isn't acting right today."

At times, it can be difficult to determine if a baby truly has CLABSI because some staphylococcal bacteria always live on a baby's skin and can contaminate the blood culture bottle, resulting in a false-positive blood culture test result. On the other hand, the blood culture test result may be negative, but the baby appears to truly have an infection. The NICU team must use their best judgment to determine which newborns need treatment and for how long.

The health care team works hard to prevent CLABSI. Good handwashing, strict sterile methods during insertion of lines, expert care during line use, and removal of catheters as soon as they are no longer needed are key to preventing infections. Central line–associated bloodstream infections are treated with IV antibiotics. Frequently, central lines must be removed to successfully treat the infection. Although most newborns recover from the infection, it is a setback in their progress and often increases the length of their hospital stay.

> 66 There's a lot of art in medicine, and sometimes different attending doctors will have different ideas about what's going on and how to address it. 99
>
> *Alex, father of **Pascal***

Preventing Hospital-Acquired Infections

Each NICU has its own policies for preventing infection. Your baby's nurse will tell you what to expect in your NICU. *Handwashing is the best way to protect your baby from a hospital-acquired infection.* Each time you come to the NICU, you will be asked to scrub your hands. Many NICUs supply alcohol-based hand sanitizer at each bedside to use before and after touching your baby.

If you or your family members have any signs of illness, consult your baby's doctor or nurse before coming to the NICU. In some cases, it may be better to stay away until you are well rather than risk exposing your baby. What is a simple cold or stomach bug for you can become a serious infection for your baby.

When your baby faces challenges, it may help to support each other as a family.
Courtesy of University of Washington Medical Center, Seattle, WA.

Problems With a Baby's Blood

Hypoglycemia

Hypoglycemia means *low blood sugar.* Your baby uses sugar (*glucose*) to produce energy. Before birth, the fetus is supplied with a constant amount of glucose across the placenta. Glucose is used by the fetus for energy and growth. During the last 3 months of pregnancy, healthy, full-term fetuses have the chance to store some glucose for use after birth. However, if the placenta was not working well, the fetus did not grow well, or the baby was born early, there may not be much glucose storage.

When the umbilical cord is cut, the glucose supply ends and the newborn has to depend on stored glucose or nutrients provided from breast milk, formula, or IV fluid. In healthy, full-term newborns, the blood glucose level falls during the first few hours after birth and then stabilizes as the body forms glucose from substances like protein and fat.

Risk of Hypoglycemia

Babies can become hypoglycemic for several reasons. Babies born to pregnant people with diabetes temporarily make too much of the hormone that lowers blood sugar (*insulin*). Babies who become cold, need resuscitation, are working hard to breathe, or are born preterm or small for gestational age can quickly use up whatever stored glucose they had, resulting in hypoglycemia.

Signs of Hypoglycemia

The common signs of hypoglycemia include tremors or jitters, irregular breathing, and floppy muscle tone. Some newborns may not have any signs, so any baby who is at risk for hypoglycemia is carefully monitored. The fastest method is to test a drop of blood from a small puncture of the baby's heel using a small glucose monitor at the baby's bedside. If the test result indicates low blood sugar, an additional sample may be sent to the laboratory for a more precise result.

Treatment of Hypoglycemia

Babies at risk of hypoglycemia and those who have mild, transient hypoglycemia may only need early and frequent feedings or temporary use of an oral gel with a high glucose content. If hypoglycemia is more significant, causes serious signs, or is persistent, it will be treated with IV fluids. Some babies have persistent, severe hypoglycemia and may need to have an IV line placed in a large blood vessel (such as an *umbilical vein catheter*) and receive IV fluids with a high concentration of sugar. Other babies may need to receive medications to raise their blood sugar level and will have additional blood tests to diagnose the cause of the hypoglycemia.

Jaundice

Red blood cells (RBCs) in newborns have a short life span. When the body breaks down old blood cells, a substance called *bilirubin* is released into the bloodstream. Before the body can dispose of the bilirubin, the liver must change the bilirubin's chemical structure so it can be removed from the baby's body in urine and stool (*bowel movements*). Before birth, the baby's bilirubin is transferred across the placenta and the pregnant person's liver does this job.

The enzyme in the baby's liver that changes bilirubin's chemical structure is not very active at birth. In other words, it takes a few days to "turn on." Until the liver can do this job, bilirubin builds up in the newborn's blood and can be seen in the baby's skin as a yellow color (*jaundice*).

Physiologic Jaundice

In most babies, bilirubin levels reach their peak toward the end of the first week and then gradually fall over the next 1 to 2 weeks. The peak level is higher in preterm newborns and may remain higher for longer. This type of jaundice is common, occurring in nearly half of full-term newborns and up to 80% of preterm newborns. It does not mean that something is wrong with your baby's liver. It is simply a result of your baby's immature liver function and is called *physiologic jaundice.* Physiologic jaundice does not require any treatment.

Hyperbilirubinemia

If the bilirubin level rises higher or faster than normal, the condition is called *hyperbilirubinemia.* Some families have an inherited blood problem that causes higher bilirubin levels. Other problems, such as infection, may alter liver function and cause a rapid increase in bilirubin levels. If your baby is at risk for hyperbilirubinemia, the bilirubin levels will be monitored closely.

Anything that causes more RBCs to break down, such as bruising during birth, increases the amount of bilirubin the liver must handle. Blood type incompatibility between the pregnant person and baby is another cause of increased RBC breakdown (see Chapter 1). When babies are not feeding, they may have difficulty removing bilirubin from their blood because bilirubin is typically excreted in their stools.

Phototherapy involves use of a blue-green light to treat hyperbilirubinemia. **Isaac** wears eye patches to protect his eyes from the light.

Eliana and her mom relax with kangaroo care during phototherapy. The box on the couch provides power to light the phototherapy blanket. The lighted phototherapy blanket is probably wrapped around Eliana's back and legs so that she and her mom are still skin-to-skin.

> ❝ Take lots of pictures and videos. They will give you strength during the hardest times when you look back. ❞
>
> *Parina, mother of **Isaac** and **Eliza***

Treatment of Hyperbilirubinemia

If the bilirubin level reaches a point that requires treatment, *phototherapy* will be started. Phototherapy involves use of blue-green light waves to change the shape of the bilirubin molecule so it can be eliminated in the baby's urine or stool without requiring the extra step in the liver. Patches are commonly placed over a baby's eyes during phototherapy to shield them from the bright light. Most newborns who require treatment for hyperbilirubinemia can be successfully treated with phototherapy.

Rarely, phototherapy cannot adequately control the bilirubin level. In this case, an *exchange transfusion* may be necessary. During this procedure, a calculated amount of the baby's blood is withdrawn through an IV line in the umbilical cord (*umbilical catheter*) and replaced with matched blood from the blood bank.

With proper management, hyperbilirubinemia causes no long-term effects. The main reason hyperbilirubinemia is treated is because bilirubin is a molecule that can cross the brain's protective barrier. If excessively high levels of bilirubin pass into the brain, it can cause a disorder called *kernicterus* and result in brain damage. Kernicterus is a very rare problem in the United States.

A Different Type of Jaundice

The common type of jaundice described previously is caused by *unconjugated bilirubin,* also called *indirect bilirubin.* A different type of jaundice is caused by *conjugated* or *direct bilirubin.* This type of jaundice is much less common and the causes are more complex. This type of hyperbilirubinemia often indicates an abnormality in liver function or a blockage in the flow of waste products leaving the liver. If your baby has conjugated hyperbilirubinemia, talk with your medical team to discuss the possible cause and treatment. Phototherapy is not typically used for this type of hyperbilirubinemia.

Neurologic Problems

Birth Depression

If blood flow into or out of the placenta is decreased during labor, the fetus may not receive enough oxygen for a period of time. When this happens, the fetal heart may have trouble pumping and it may not be able to provide enough blood flow and oxygen to other cells in the body. The baby may be born limp, not breathing, and with a low heart rate. This is called *birth depression.*

The lack of blood flow in the fetus is known as *ischemia.* The cells have low oxygen (the cells are *hypoxic*), cannot work properly, and begin to produce waste products in the form of acids. These acids build up, a condition called *acidemia,* and can damage many of the body's cells. If birth depression from lack of blood flow and oxygen results in abnormal brain function, the condition is called *hypoxic-ischemic encephalopathy (HIE).*

Causes of Birth Depression

Anything that interferes with blood and oxygen flowing into or out of the placenta can cause birth depression. Problems with placental blood flow can occur because of infection, abnormal placental development, separation of the placenta from the uterus before birth, or a placenta that is not working well. All of these things can influence oxygen supply to the fetus.

The oxygen supply to the fetus is temporarily decreased during labor contractions; this is a normal and expected part of the labor process. However, sometimes contractions occur that are unusually strong, too close together, or last an unusually long time. The umbilical cord carries blood and oxygen to the baby from the placenta and it can become squeezed during contractions if it is wrapped tightly around the baby; during a very difficult delivery; or if it slips into the birth canal before the baby (*prolapsed cord*).

Factors That Can Cause Birth Depression

- Separation of the placenta from the uterine wall before birth (placental abruption)
- Squeezing (compression) of the umbilical cord during labor and delivery, a cord tightened around the baby's neck (nuchal cord), a cord trapped below the baby in the birth canal (prolapsed cord)
- Prolonged or difficult delivery
- Unusual presentation during vaginal birth, such as buttocks first or legs first (breech presentation)
- Severe infection in the pregnant person or fetus
- High or severely low blood pressure in the pregnant person
- Lack of oxygen to the pregnant person (for example, due to acute asthma, severe pneumonia, or seizures)
- Umbilical cord accident (for example, a cord that ties in a knot in the uterus, a cord that tangles with a twin)
- Severe injury to the pregnant person (for example, from a car crash)
- Severe lack of red blood cells (anemia) in the fetus due to infection, damage to the red blood cells, or bleeding into the pregnant person's circulation or into a twin

Preventing Birth Depression

The obstetric team will try to identify pregnancies at risk for problems with placental function and help before the baby is affected. If the pregnant person has high blood pressure or diabetes, for example, or if the fetus is not growing or gaining weight, prenatal testing with ultrasound or electronic monitoring of the baby's heart rate may be done to make sure the fetus is in good condition. Labor may be induced or cesarean birth planned if the obstetric team decides that waiting for labor to start on its own could endanger the baby. During labor and delivery, fetal heart rate monitoring is one tool that can help detect problems. The goal is to deliver the baby before problems develop from poor placental function but not so early as to cause major problems of prematurity.

Severe birth depression is an unusual problem, with most factors being outside anyone's control. Birth depression is often unknown until a pregnant individual presents with a problem such as decreased fetal movement or continuous severe belly pain. During the examination, the nurse or physician may detect a fetal heart rate that is too fast (*tachycardic*), too slow (*bradycardic*), or too steady (does not change in response to fetal movement or stimulation). The nurse or physician may find significant vaginal bleeding, abdominal tenderness, the umbilical cord in the birth canal (*prolapsed umbilical cord*), or other signs of potential fetal distress such as the presence of meconium (baby's first stool) in the amniotic fluid (see the Meconium Aspiration Syndrome [MAS] section earlier in this chapter).

Mild Birth Depression

Babies who have only mild birth depression may recover quickly after birth. They may briefly need additional oxygen or breathing support for several minutes until they begin breathing well on their own. After stabilization, babies with mild depression will be monitored. Sometimes, feeding is delayed to allow the bowel to rest and recover from a possible interruption in adequate oxygen supply.

Severe Birth Depression

Babies with severe birth depression may need more complex care after birth. The medical team may need to place a temporary breathing tube in the baby's windpipe (endotracheal intubation), assist breathing, do chest compressions to help the baby's heart pump blood, and give emergency medications.

Newborns with severe birth depression often need help breathing with a ventilator. Occasionally, the blood vessels in the lungs don't relax properly, leading to a condition called PPHN (see the Persistent Pulmonary Hypertension of the Newborn [PPHN] section earlier in this chapter). They may have decreased heart function and need medications to help their heart pump with more strength. They need careful management of glucose and fluids, especially if the kidneys have been injured by lack of blood flow and oxygen. Brain injury often leads to seizures during the first days after birth. Babies with severe birth depression are often very ill and have major complications, and some do not survive.

Complications of Birth Depression

- Seizures
- Brain injury
- Low blood pressure
- Respiratory distress
- Kidney injury
- Bowel injury
- Low blood sugar
- Bleeding

Hypoxic-Ischemic Encephalopathy

Birth depression can result in HIE. As described earlier, HIE is caused by lack of oxygen in the blood (*hypoxia*) and reduced blood flow to the brain (*ischemia*). These events lead to brain dysfunction (*encephalopathy*).

Hypoxic-ischemic encephalopathy is often divided into 3 stages: mild, moderate, and severe. Most often, mild HIE has a good outcome, and treatment in the newborn period is only supportive, as described previously. Moderate and severe HIE continue to be important causes of acute brain injury and may benefit from additional therapy.

Therapeutic Hypothermia

Therapeutic hypothermia, also called *cooling,* is a safe and effective treatment for babies born within a few weeks of their due date (term, post term, and late preterm) with moderate or severe HIE. Lowering the baby's body temperature after birth appears to reduce the amount of damage to brain cells and improve the chance of survival without major disabilities. It appears to be most effective for babies with moderate HIE, but is also offered to babies with more severe HIE.

Babies must meet certain conditions to qualify for therapeutic hypothermia, and it appears to be most effective if it is started within the first few hours after birth. Therapeutic hypothermia is provided in specialized NICUs, which often requires rapid transport of eligible babies to a NICU that can provide this treatment so cooling can be started in time.

The 2 methods currently being used are *selective head cooling* and *whole body cooling.* For selective head cooling, the baby wears a special cooling cap. For whole body cooling, the baby lays on a cooling mattress. With either method, the baby's temperature is kept between 33°C and 34°C (91.4°F to 93.2°F) for 72 hours. During cooling, the baby's heart rate often decreases, but as long as the blood pressure and oxygen saturation are stable, no assistance is needed. At the end of the cooling period, the baby is gradually rewarmed.

Outcome for Babies With Birth Depression

Most babies recover well from mild or moderate birth depression, but some will have long-term disabilities, such as problems thinking, seeing, hearing, or walking. Even with hypothermia treatment, many newborns with severe HIE will die or survive with disabilities. It may be very difficult for doctors to predict how well your baby will do until months or even years later. Sometimes, magnetic resonance imaging (MRI) of the brain in the newborn period can provide some clues about the baby's likelihood of having disabilities.

Seizures

Seizures occur when there is a sudden surge of electrical signals in the brain. Seizures can be a sign of brain injury or irritation. They may appear as jerking movements of the arms or legs, stiffening of an extremity or arching of the back, facial twitching, head turning, or repetitive movements of the eyes, lips, or tongue. A pause in breathing (*apnea*) and sudden changes in blood pressure may also occur. At times, seizures can be very subtle and hard to detect. Babies can have normal jittery movements that are not seizures. Normal jittery movements stop when a hand is placed on the baby's trembling arms or legs; however, seizure activity does not.

Causes of Seizures

Often, no cause can be found. Seizures may result from brain injury, infection, chemical imbalances in the blood (for example, low blood sugar, low calcium), bleeding in the brain or surrounding tissues, swelling of the brain, or malformation of the brain.

Diagnosis of Seizures

If the NICU team suspects seizures, they will study your baby's brain waves using a painless test called an *electroencephalogram* (*EEG*). This test involves placing sensors on the baby's scalp and recording the electrical activity in the brain. Seizures appear as abnormal patterns of electrical activity on the brain-wave tracing.

Other tests that may be done include

▸ An ultrasound of the brain to look for bleeding or unusual brain structure

▸ Computed tomographic (CT) scan or magnetic resonance imaging (MRI) to look for bleeding, swelling, or unusual brain structure or unusual blood vessels

▸ Blood tests to look for chemical imbalances (for example, glucose, sodium, calcium, acids)

▸ Blood and spinal fluid tests to look for infection

A doctor specializing in disorders of the brain and nervous system (*neurologist*) may also examine your baby and help the NICU team manage your baby's problems.

Treatment for Seizures

The first priority is to treat any underlying cause of the seizure, such as low blood sugar. Seizures are treated with medications that decrease the brain's electrical activity. The duration of treatment varies from just a few days to several months or longer, depending on the underlying problem and frequency of seizures.

Potential Outcome for a Baby With Seizures

The outcome for a baby who has seizures depends on what is causing the seizures, the presence of brain injury from the underlying cause, the severity of seizures, and the type of seizures. Many babies recover completely, with no signs of brain damage, especially if the seizures are brief and infrequent. Seizures caused by severe birth depression or serious brain injury may persist for a longer period and are associated with a higher risk of learning disabilities, developmental delays, and neurologic abnormalities. Follow-up visits with the neurologist or developmental specialists may be needed to evaluate your baby's progress over a long period.

Stay Informed

This chapter has explained many of the serious medical problems that can bring a baby to the NICU. This information is intended to give you a basic understanding of each problem but does not replace discussions with your baby's NICU team.

Keep in mind that just as each baby is unique, so is each NICU. There are different approaches to treating many of these problems, and new discoveries are helping to improve the care of babies every day.

Colson

Born at 35 weeks

• • • • • • • • • • • •

Colson received his NICU care in a children's hospital.

We found out around 16 weeks of gestation that Colson had an abdominal wall abnormality. We were very worried about his prognosis and weren't sure what to do. At 23 weeks' gestation we had confirmation through a CT scan that Colson had a giant omphalocele.* We met with several doctors in our health care system and decided to get a second opinion. We were referred to a children's hospital where we met with pediatric surgeons, neonatologists, and genetic specialists. The information and references we received from the doctors helped us decide that we would continue to manage my pregnancy within our local health care system because it was closer to home, but deliver Colson at a hospital farther away that was connected to the children's hospital where he would receive intensive care.

We had already set a date for a scheduled cesarean section when Colson decided to make an early debut at 35 weeks of gestation. We drove to the hospital about an hour away from home and I had an emergency cesarean section. Colson was immediately admitted to the NICU at the children's hospital.

Colson remained in the NICU for 7 months before he could come home. Since Colson was premature with an omphalocele, his lungs were underdeveloped. The NICU staff was very supportive and informative, and they valued our opinions as parents when making medical decisions regarding Colson's health.

Colson spent 7 months in the hospital, where the NICU team became part of Colson's family.

Since we lived so far away and had 2 other kids at home (as well as our own restaurant business), only one of us could be with Colson on a daily basis. The NICU staff made sure that we were comfortable and that Colson was getting the care he needed so that he could come home to his family. During our 7 months in the NICU, we felt like we made everlasting memories and relationships with his nurses, physician assistants, doctors, respiratory therapists, occupational therapists, physical therapists, and everyone else who cared for Colson. It was like we made a new family in the NICU.

* An omphalocele is a defect in the abdominal wall in which the intestines and possibly other abdominal organs (stomach, liver, spleen) are contained in a sac outside of the body, within the umbilical cord.

When Colson was finally ready to come home, we were given training, supplies, and everything else needed to care for him. Colson also joined the Little Victors League offered at the children's hospital. It is a team that works alongside Colson's caregivers and offers help with his outpatient care. The children's hospital went above and beyond for Colson and our needs. We are absolutely grateful for the care that we received for our little warrior.

Jewel and Soua, parents of Colson

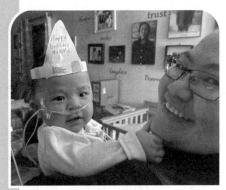

Colson came home in time to celebrate his mother's birthday.

Holland
&
Eden

Born at 24 weeks, 3 days

Mom's hands comfort Holland.

Eden in her early NICU days.

Holland and Eden were born at 24 weeks 3 days' gestation, weighing just over 1 pound each. At the time of their birth, there was no infection, no abnormalities, and never an explanation for why they came so early. They were born with their eyes still fused shut and skin so thin that you could see through it. They were perfectly formed and, to us, already beautiful.

Our girls spent the first 110 days of their lives in the NICU. During that time, we had some very long and very sad days. Both girls were transferred for patent ductus arteriosus (PDA) ligation surgery on their hearts. They both underwent laser surgery on their eyes for retinopathy of prematurity. We lived through more than one infection, one which Holland almost didn't survive. Both had some degree of bleeding in the brain. Both needed a lot of coaxing to learn to eat and grow. We experienced a great deal of guilt, grief, and devastation.

Our time in the NICU was also filled with small moments of happiness and even times of great joy. I clearly remember the nurse who asked if I wanted to hold each baby for the first time and how much work they would do to get us ready for kangaroo care. I remember the care with which they taught us how to touch our babies, how to change their tiny diapers, how to take their temperatures. I remember the doctors giving hugs and high fives when Holland's platelets finally went back up following a nasty infection. I remember them listening to our endless questions and sitting down with us to draw diagrams to help us understand complicated medical issues, never annoyed by our incessant attention to detail. I remember the encouragement they gave me in pumping and attempting to breastfeed and how they kept me motivated by always oohing and aahing over the calorie content of my milk. I will be forever grateful to the doctors and nurses who touched our lives at that time and took such good care of our family.

Unfortunately, our struggles did not end when we left the NICU. We went home with oxygen, monitors, and countless doctor appointments for the first 6 months. Holland has had ongoing issues with asthma, vision, mild cerebral palsy (CP), attention, and anxiety. She has had multiple eye surgeries and has been hospitalized several times with pneumonia and respiratory illnesses. She did not start walking until after she was 2, and still struggles to keep up with her peers in physical activities. Eating and growing continue to be a challenge, and she did not hit 50 pounds until this past summer.

Eden has more severe CP and is unable to stand or walk. She uses a power wheelchair as her main source of mobility. We spend a lot of time and money on equipment and therapies to help her achieve her potential. In addition to the CP, Eden was diagnosed with profound bilateral hearing loss at 6 months of age and underwent her first cochlear implant surgery when she was 14 months old. She received her second implant at age 9. She also underwent vocal cord reinnervation surgery to help improve her vocal quality from a paralyzed vocal cord. Between the 2 girls, we have been through 12 surgeries.

A take-home baby! Holland and Eden welcome new baby sister Violet.

While I feel like it is important for people to be aware of the ongoing issues that extremely premature infants face, I really hate listing their disabilities or medical issues when describing them. Terms like "chronic lung disease," or "profound hearing loss," or "cerebral palsy" do not give you any insight into the amazing people that they are becoming. I'd rather tell you about how Eden's smile lights up a room and how Holland's giggles are completely contagious. They are both voracious readers. Holland is passionate about video games, Pokémon, Skylanders, and stand-up comedy. She loves stories of all kinds and still loves to pretend. She also loves exploring nature, swimming, and collecting trinkets.

Eden loves adventure, from snorkeling to roller coasters to big cities, and pictures herself traveling the world, next stop…Tokyo. She loves Japanese manga and learning about Asian culture. She is a blossoming foodie who will try anything and shares her Dad's appetite for spicy mussels. She also loves having big discussions about everything from health care to history, world religions to disability rights. They both enrich our lives and bring us such joy every day.

I am not a person who believes that everything happens for a reason. What I *do* believe is that when bad things happen, we can become better people because of them. We can learn and grow from them. I am a better person because of my kids and what they have gone through following their traumatic birth. I do not take life for granted. I don't sweat the small stuff. I have learned to appreciate every step of progress they make, no matter how small it may seem. I am better able to support people who are going through similar circumstances. I am more compassionate and a better advocate for my children's needs. In addition to all of that, I have had the opportunity to meet so many incredible people who I would never have known otherwise, and my life is richer because of them. **Read more about Holland and Eden in "Where Are They Now?" in the Appendix.**

Billie, mother of Holland & Eden

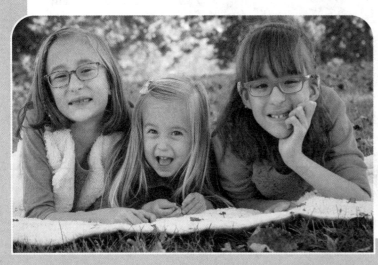

Holland, Violet, and Eden.

CHAPTER 5

Your Preterm Baby

"

I asked my OB what could be
done to stop the contractions and
her answer caught me off guard.
I was fully dilated, she told me, and there
was no stopping this baby. Our world was
completely rocked. Within minutes, our
mighty Alexander was born at just
26 weeks' gestation.

*Stacy, mother of **Alex***

"

More than 365,000 babies are born prematurely (preterm) in the United States each year. Recently, the overall rate of preterm birth has slightly decreased, but we still expect about 1 in 10 babies in the United States to be born too soon. The risk for preterm birth remains higher, and has slightly increased, for Black and American Indian/Alaska Native babies. Preterm birth can be related to problems with the pregnant person's health or a problem with the growing fetus, but about half the time, preterm labor happens for unknown reasons. For more information see **https://www.cdc.gov/ reproductivehealth/maternalinfanthealth/pretermbirth.htm.**

Please use this QR code to go directly to www.cdc.gov/ reproductivehealth/ maternalinfanthealth/ pretermbirth.htm.

By the time your baby is born, even if delivery occurs well before your due date, all the major body systems have been formed, but they are immature and still developing. The organ systems may not function the same way they would in a full-term newborn and are at risk of injury or abnormal development.

Your baby's neonatal intensive care unit (NICU) team knows the wide range of problems that can affect preterm newborns. They can recognize early signs of developing problems and take steps that keep little problems from becoming a crisis. Although preterm babies may be *at risk* of developing the problems described in this chapter, it does not mean that all preterm babies *will* develop these problems. Talk with your NICU team about any concerns you have for your preterm baby.

How Does a Preterm Baby Look?

A preterm baby's appearance is related to their gestational age at birth. In fact, by examining your baby's physical features, the NICU team can estimate your baby's gestational age within a couple of weeks. This examination is called a *Ballard score*. The information in the box titled "Physical Features of a Very Preterm Baby" describes features of a very preterm baby. Infants who are more mature will have fewer of these features.

Physical Features of a Very Preterm Baby

- Fused (closed) eyelids
- Thin, smooth skin
- Visible veins under the skin, especially over the tummy
- Flat or invisible nipples
- Absent or decrease in fine hair (*lanugo*) over the baby's back and neck
- Smooth soles of the feet
- Soft, thin ears that do not spring back when folded
- No testes yet positioned in the scrotum (boys)
- Little fat in the vaginal labia (girls)
- Flexible joints at the hips and knees
- Limp muscle tone

At 22 weeks and 5 days of gestation, **Abel** has the shiny skin of an extremely preterm newborn. The "nest" of rolled blankets keeps his arms and legs in a flexed position to promote normal growth and development.

Why Are Preterm Babies at Greater Risk of Complications?

Babies who are more preterm have a higher risk of complications and will likely require a higher level of care. Preterm babies are at a higher risk because they are born with

- Immature lungs and a decreased amount of *surfactant,* a slippery soap-like substance that keeps the tiny air sacs in their lungs from collapsing as the baby breathes in and out
- Weak muscles that make it difficult to breathe
- Thin skin and reduced fat that put the baby at risk for a low body temperature (*hypothermia*)
- Immature tissues that are easily damaged if exposed to too much oxygen
- Immature immune system that puts the baby at risk of infection
- Immature blood vessels in the brain that are easily damaged, thereby causing bleeding
- Less stored glucose that puts the baby at risk for low blood sugar (*hypoglycemia*)
- Smaller blood volume and a frequent need for blood tests that put the baby at risk for a reduced number of red blood cells (*anemia*)

Problems Affecting the Preterm Baby's Lungs

The lungs are responsible for maintaining the correct amount of oxygen and carbon dioxide in your baby's body. Too much or too little of either gas is unhealthy.

When we breathe in, air travels into the lungs through a series of tubes that gradually get smaller until air reaches tiny sacs called *alveoli* (similar to branching of trees). The alveoli are surrounded by small blood vessels called *capillaries* that allow oxygen to move into the bloodstream to be carried to the rest of the body. Carbon dioxide, the waste gas made by the body, is brought to the alveoli of the lungs through the bloodstream and is exhaled when we breathe out.

Preterm babies may have difficulty with many of the lungs' functions. These problems may begin in the delivery room and include difficulty starting breathing, keeping their lungs open, or controlling the normal rate of breathing. They may take shallow breaths, not breathe (*apnea*), or breathe too fast (*tachypnea*).

Breathing Problems at Birth

Before birth, a baby's lungs are full of fluid and do not provide oxygen to the body. Instead, oxygen moves from the pregnant person's blood through the placenta and umbilical cord to the fetus. At birth, babies must quickly begin breathing, inflate their lungs with air, remove the fluid from their lungs, use their lungs to carry oxygen to the blood, and use their heart to pump it to the rest of their body.

Although many preterm babies cry at birth and require little help from the NICU team, more than half of babies delivered before 33 weeks' gestation have trouble breathing. The medical team member caring for your baby at birth may use a face mask and a mechanical device to assist your baby's first breaths. Some babies may need to have a breathing tube placed in their throat and advanced to their windpipe (*endotracheal intubation*) to provide more assistance with breathing.

> " He was having a lot of trouble breathing on his own, so he was going to be intubated. It was at that exact moment that I realized how serious this whole situation was. That moment defined me as a new mom of a preemie. "
>
> *Marnie, mother of **Kellan***

Respiratory Distress Syndrome (RDS)

Respiratory distress syndrome (*RDS*) is the most common lung condition affecting preterm babies. It mostly affects babies born before 35 weeks' gestation, but occasionally more mature newborns can develop RDS. The earlier a baby is born, the more likely RDS will be diagnosed, and the more severe the disease is likely to be.

Respiratory distress syndrome is caused by immaturity of the baby's chest and lungs and a decreased amount of *surfactant*. Surfactant is a soap-like substance made in the lungs that coats the inside of the tiny breathing sacs (*alveoli*) and helps to keep them open as the baby breathes in and out. Without enough surfactant, the alveoli tend to collapse between breaths. If the alveoli collapse, the baby has to do extra work to reopen them with each breath. Over time, the alveoli may not open enough, causing oxygen levels to decrease and the carbon dioxide level to increase in the baby's blood.

Each baby's lungs mature at a different rate. Surfactant production begins around the 24th week of gestation, but the system is not fully developed until 34 to 36 weeks. Giving corticosteroids to the pregnant person before preterm delivery is safe and can help speed up the production of surfactant in the fetal lungs.

Signs of RDS

Preterm babies may show signs of RDS within minutes after birth, or they may develop breathing problems in the first few hours after birth. You may notice your baby is breathing fast (*tachypnea*) or working hard to breathe. The newborn may have labored breathing that causes the skin and muscles between the ribs or just below the rib cage to pull in during breaths (*retractions*) or make a moaning sound (*grunting*) when breathing out. Blue color around your

Auggie follows a fairly typical pathway through respiratory support devices.

For several weeks after his very preterm birth, **Auggie** needed endotracheal intubation and a ventilator to help him breathe. Not all preterm babies need a ventilator after birth.

When **Auggie** could breathe well on his own, he used a nasal cannula to deliver CPAP to lessen the work of breathing.

When **Auggie** grew stronger, he graduated from CPAP and used a nasal cannula to provide a gentle flow of air/oxygen.

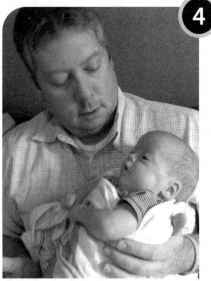

Finallly, **Auggie** no longer needed extra air flow or oxygen through the nasal cannula and is shown here with his proud father.

baby's lips (*cyanosis*) or a pale and blotchy (*mottled*) appearance of the skin may develop. If your baby is working hard to breathe and gets tired, an uneven breathing rate may occur and pauses in breathing (*apnea*) may be seen.

> " You don't realize how strong you have to be to be a preemie parent, a NICU parent. These babies give us the emotional ride of our lives. "
>
> *Lisa, mother of* **Frankie**

Diagnosis of RDS

If RDS is suspected, your baby's NICU team may order a chest x-ray (*radiograph*) and a blood test called a *blood gas*. The chest x-rays of babies with RDS often have a hazy white and grainy appearance. In some NICUs, an ultrasound of the lungs may be used to look for signs of RDS. The baby's blood gas test may show a low oxygen level and a high carbon dioxide level. There is, however, no perfect test to diagnose RDS. For example, the x-ray of a newborn with RDS looks a lot like an x-ray of a newborn with pneumonia. Respiratory distress syndrome is diagnosed by evaluating all the diagnostic test results in combination with the baby's history, physical examination findings, and progress over the first days after birth.

Treatment of RDS: Continuous Positive Airway Pressure (CPAP) and Surfactant

The best options for treating RDS continue to be an area of active research. Babies with mild RDS may only require additional oxygen through tubing connected to small plastic prongs called a *nasal cannula.*

Babies with more serious RDS may receive breathing support through CPAP. Nasal CPAP maintains air pressure, and sometimes additional oxygen, in the baby's lungs through prongs placed in the nose or through a small mask placed over the nose (see Chapter 3). Nasal CPAP helps to stabilize the baby's chest wall and alveoli and prevent them from collapsing between breaths. Although CPAP helps to keep the lungs open, the machine does not provide any breaths, so babies receiving CPAP must take their own breaths. In some NICUs, babies who do not reliably take their own breaths, or need more breathing support, will receive breaths from a mechanical ventilator into the baby's nose through the CPAP prongs or mask. This is called *noninvasive positive-pressure ventilation* (*NIPPV*).

Babies with the most serious RDS may need additional surfactant administered into their lungs and breathing assistance from a mechanical ventilator while their lungs mature. If mechanical ventilation is needed, a breathing tube (*endotracheal tube*) is temporarily placed in the baby's windpipe (*trachea*) in a procedure called *intubation* (see Chapter 1).

Frequently, preterm babies with respiratory distress are treated with CPAP first. If the baby's breathing worsens, the baby is intubated and surfactant is given through the breathing tube. Sometimes, the endotracheal tube is removed immediately after surfactant is administered, and the baby's breathing support returns to CPAP. Sometimes, the baby needs to stay intubated and receive breathing support from a ventilator for a period of time. In some NICUs, surfactant will be given through a thin catheter instead of an endotracheal tube, and the baby will stay on CPAP. In either case, depending on the baby's response, 1 or 2 more doses of surfactant may be given. The goal is to decrease the amount of additional oxygen needed and the time spent on a ventilator.

If your baby will be born preterm, ask a member of the NICU team what you can expect regarding CPAP, NIPPV, surfactant, and mechanical ventilation.

Allison needed CPAP at birth.

At 4 days old, **Reece** no longer needed the steady airway pressure from CPAP and graduated to a nasal cannula with a gentle flow of air/oxygen only.

Abel, born at 22 weeks and 5 days, was intubated for 110 days after his birth.

Air Leaks

Air leaks were described in Chapter 4. They occur when breathing sacs (*alveoli*) rupture, allowing air to leak into the tissue surrounding the lung. Preterm babies are at higher risk for air leaks because babies with RDS have stiff lungs that don't open and close as easily as healthy lungs. When a baby with stiff lungs breathes or receives help from CPAP or a ventilator, 1 or more of the thin-walled alveoli can rupture. In preterm babies with RDS, surfactant helps decrease the risk of air leaks. If air becomes trapped between the lung and rib cage (*pneumothorax*), the air may be removed with a needle or a thin plastic or silicone tube (*chest tube*) attached to a vacuum system (*suction*).

Pulmonary interstitial emphysema (PIE) is a special type of air leak in which air becomes trapped in many small spaces and cannot be removed with a needle or chest tube. Babies with PIE often require gentle ventilator support until their lungs heal. The NICU team may allow the baby to have lower blood oxygen levels or higher carbon dioxide levels temporarily to decrease the ventilator pressure while the lungs are healing. In some cases, a special ventilator (*high-frequency ventilator*) that delivers tiny breaths at a high rate of speed may be used (see Chapter 4).

Bronchopulmonary Dysplasia (BPD)

Bronchopulmonary dysplasia (*BPD*), also called *chronic lung disease* (*CLD*) of preterm babies, is a lung disease occurring mostly in babies born between 22 and 32 weeks' gestation. The definition of BPD varies but is often described as a preterm baby born at less than 32 weeks' gestation who has required additional oxygen (more than 21% oxygen) for at least 4 weeks and continues to require oxygen at what would have been 36 weeks' gestational age.

Researchers are still trying to understand exactly what causes BPD and how it can be prevented. Babies with BPD have fewer and larger alveoli and fewer blood vessels surrounding their alveoli. This means the lungs have a smaller area to use for breathing. In addition, some babies with BPD may have thickened, swollen, and scarred airways within their lungs. This damage might have been caused by injury and inflammation from repeated opening and closing of the tiny alveoli while the baby received respiratory support. Inflammation is part of the body's response to an injury and can promote healing, but when inflammation gets out of control, it can damage the body.

Risk Factors for BPD

Researchers still do not know why some preterm babies without any risk factors develop BPD. Genetics and family history may play a role because inherited genes can affect how your baby's lungs respond to an injury.

Overall, BPD occurs in approximately 20% to 40% of babies who are born at 27 to 29 weeks' gestation; the rate increases to greater than 50% at lower gestational ages, but the rate of BPD varies widely among different hospitals. Some of the risk factors for BPD are listed in the box titled "Risk Factors for Bronchopulmonary Dysplasia."

Risk Factors for Bronchopulmonary Dysplasia

- Lower gestational age at birth
- Infection of the amniotic fluid before birth (*chorioamnionitis*)
- Severe respiratory distress syndrome (RDS)
- Prolonged mechanical ventilation
- Pneumonia
- Poor nutrition
- Excess fluid in the lung

Diagnosis and Treatment of BPD

Babies with RDS usually begin to improve after several days to a week of treatment. Newborns who develop BPD often have more severe RDS at first, are slow to improve, or may begin to improve and then stop making progress. Chest x-rays may show a hazy, streaky, or bubbly appearance in the lungs.

The goal of BPD treatment is to allow the newborn's lung to heal while new, undamaged lung tissue develops. Treatment for BPD includes administering additional oxygen and/or pressure into the lungs, supplying good nutrition with enough calories to promote growth, and avoiding excess fluid in the lungs. Additional vitamin A in your baby's diet may help prevent BPD. Other medications may be used to help improve your baby's lung function, but none have been proven to prevent BPD or change its course. Medications such as furosemide (Lasix), spironolactone (Aldactone), and chlorothiazide (Diuril) help babies make additional urine and also may help decrease the amount of fluid in the lungs. Babies with BPD may produce additional mucus and have episodes of wheezing or narrowing of the air passages (*bronchospasm*). Inhaled medications to relax the airway might be used if your baby experiences episodes of wheezing.

Some babies with BPD have sudden changes in their vital signs, commonly called *spells or exacerbations,* especially when they become upset. During these episodes, the baby may become blue (*cyanotic*), have a low heart rate (*bradycardia*), and have a lower oxygen level (*oxygen desaturation* or *desat*). Sometimes, these events occur at a predictable time each day or during specific activities (for example, when your baby tries to pass a stool). Parents and the medical team can often identify the triggers that begin these episodes and learn how to prevent or stop them.

Babies with severe BPD may require treatment with a steroid to decrease the inflammation in their lungs. Although steroids given to pregnant individuals before preterm birth are safe and helpful, steroids are not routinely given to preterm babies after birth. They may offer short-term benefits by allowing babies to wean off a mechanical ventilator more quickly; however, they have some short-term risks and may interfere with normal brain and lung development. If your baby's team decides that steroids may be beneficial for your baby, they will discuss this with you.

Complications of BPD

Bronchopulmonary dysplasia is different for every baby. Many babies who need help breathing will have mild or moderate BPD. Mild BPD can mean that your baby requires oxygen for a month or longer but is able to go home without extra oxygen or medications. Babies with moderate BPD may need to go home with oxygen for a time, and others may require home oxygen for several months. Babies with the most severe BPD may require a prolonged hospital stay, and may even go home with a ventilator to support their breathing.

Babies with BPD often have difficulty feeding by mouth. They may not tolerate having things placed in their mouth, called *oral aversion*. Some babies with BPD may have slow emptying from their stomach, and feedings may flow backward into their food pipe (*esophagus*). This backward flow is called *reflux*. Physical therapists, occupational therapists, and speech and language pathologists may help the NICU team develop a treatment plan for babies with BPD who have difficulty with feeding.

Bronchopulmonary dysplasia is a chronic disease that can take months or, occasionally, years to resolve. Because your baby could miss the normal stages of infant growth, your baby's nurse or therapist will work with you and your baby on a variety of exercises and activities designed to promote your baby's best possible growth and development.

At birth, preterm babies have only a small fraction of the alveoli they will have when they are grown. The lungs continue to grow, and new alveoli develop for many years. Most babies with BPD show gradual improvement in their lung function after discharge but may have some abnormal lung function for years. They may not be able to deal with pollution in the air and should not be exposed to tobacco smoke. Babies with BPD have an increased risk of developing asthma and pneumonia. If they develop a respiratory infection like a cold or flu (*influenza*), they may become very ill and require rehospitalization. Before discharge, your baby may receive an injection (palivizumab [Synagis]) to help prevent complications from a common viral infection called *RSV* (*respiratory syncytial virus*) that occurs during the fall and winter (see Chapter 8). It is important for everyone who comes into contact with your baby to wash their hands and get a flu vaccination, and follow current guidelines for COVID vaccination (see Chapter 8).

Apnea of Prematurity

Even though fetuses do not use their lungs for actual breathing, they do make breathing movements before birth. This breathing isn't continuous and doesn't have a regular pattern. After birth, babies must develop a regular breathing pattern, even when they are sleeping, to maintain a constant supply of oxygen. Breathing patterns are controlled by a timing mechanism in the baby's brain, and the timing mechanism is not fully mature until a baby is close to full term.

Preterm babies often have irregular, or uneven, breathing patterns with episodes of shallow breathing or pauses. A prolonged breathing pause is called *apnea*. Apnea is a common problem of prematurity, occurring in 25% of all preterm babies and in more than 80% of babies weighing less than 1,000 g (about 2 lb 3 oz) at birth. When short pauses occur several times in a row, it is called *periodic breathing*. This pattern is common, especially during sleep, even among healthy term babies, and may last for many weeks after birth.

When preterm babies have apnea, their heart rate may slow, and their blood oxygen level may decrease. Slowing of the heart rate is called *bradycardia* (*bradys*) and decreases in oxygen saturation are called *desaturations* (*desats*). The NICU team may call these events *As and Bs* for *apneas and bradycardias* or *A-B-Ds* for *apneas, bradycardias, and desaturations.*

Management of Apnea of Prematurity

Babies at risk for apnea have an electronic monitor that tracks their heart and breathing rates. They may also be monitored with a pulse oximeter that tracks their blood oxygen saturation using a light that shines on their skin. Alarms go off when the heart rate, breathing rate, or oxygen saturation falls below an acceptable level for a certain period (see Chapter 3).

Apnea can be very frightening for parents, but many apneic periods end on their own and the baby begins to breathe again. If the baby does not resume breathing after a brief period of time, the medical team member may gently rub the baby's side or foot to encourage breathing (often called a *stimulation* or *stim)*. Sometimes, the caregiver also needs to give the baby extra oxygen. If the baby doesn't start breathing after stimulation or the heart rate remains low, the baby may receive additional oxygen or several assisted breaths with a face mask. Babies with frequent apnea that leads to bradycardia and desaturation may require medication, CPAP, NIPPV, or extra airflow from a nasal cannula. *Caffeine* is a medicine, given intravenously or by mouth, that stimulates the brain's breathing center and may help to normalize the baby's breathing pattern.

As the baby matures, apnea of prematurity gradually improves and finally disappears. Apnea of prematurity resolves in most preterm babies before they go home. Once apnea of prematurity resolves, it does not come back. Very preterm babies, delivered before 28 weeks' gestation, may not have fully mature breathing control until several weeks after their due date. A small number of preterm babies may require home apnea monitoring after discharge. If apnea persists at the time your baby is approaching discharge, the NICU team will discuss this with you.

Apnea of prematurity is not the same as sudden infant death syndrome (SIDS; also called *crib death*) and is not a risk factor for SIDS. The cause of SIDS is unknown. Strategies for reducing the risk of SIDS are found in Chapter 9.

Treatment Options for Apnea of Prematurity

- Careful monitoring until the baby outgrows apnea
- Caffeine
- CPAP, NIPPV, or airflow from a nasal cannula

Obstructive Apnea

Obstructive apnea occurs when the baby is trying to breathe but the airway becomes blocked. Preterm babies have low muscle tone in the upper throat, making the airway more likely to become blocked. During sleep, the airway may partially collapse and block air movement into the lungs. Obstructive apnea may also occur while a baby is being fed or held if the head falls too far forward or backward and closes the airway. It is common for preterm babies to have both obstructive apnea and apnea of prematurity (*central apnea*).

Problems Affecting the Preterm Baby's Blood

Anemia

Anemia means there is a decrease in the number of red blood cells (RBCs) in a baby's blood. Red blood cells are the part of blood that carries oxygen. The NICU team often estimates the number of RBCs by using a blood test that measures the *hemoglobin* level or *hematocrit*.

Causes of Anemia

Anemia is a common problem and has multiple causes. Preterm babies are at risk of developing anemia because their blood cells have a shorter life span than those in children and adults, and their body has a limited ability to make new blood cells. In total, babies weighing 1,500 g (3 lb 5 oz) have approximately 4 oz of blood in their bodies. Blood may be lost during birth because of a problem with the placenta or umbilical cord, or internal bleeding may cause sudden, severe blood loss. During the first few weeks after birth, blood may be lost if a baby requires frequent laboratory tests. A common cause of anemia is a combination of blood losses from laboratory tests and a decrease in blood production called *anemia of prematurity*.

> " Abel had a great NICU team. We got to know a lot of doctors who rotated in and out of the NICU, but it's so important to forge relationships with the nurse practitioners and the nurses who are there for the long haul. The consistency was there, and month after month getting to know them and how they care for and know my son made a world of difference. "
>
> *Shana, mother of **Abel***

Anemia of Prematurity

Anemia of prematurity occurs because RBC production temporarily stops after birth. A hormone called *erythropoietin* (*EPO*) is made in your baby's liver and kidney. Erythropoietin stimulates RBC production in the baby's bone marrow. Shortly after birth, EPO production stops and the bone marrow stops making RBCs. The baby's hemoglobin level gradually decreases over several weeks, reaching its lowest value between 4 and 10 weeks after birth. Eventually, the hemoglobin reaches a level at which EPO is secreted again and RBC production resumes. This process occurs even in full-term babies; however, it occurs earlier, lasts longer, and is more severe in preterm babies.

Diagnosis of Anemia

If anemia occurs very suddenly because of rapid blood loss, babies may have signs of shock, with low blood pressure, fast heart rate, weak pulses, pale or ashen gray skin color, and respiratory distress. Anemia of prematurity causes a more gradual decrease in RBCs. It may cause no signs at all, or babies' skin and gums may gradually develop a pale color. Some babies with anemia of prematurity demonstrate poor growth, decreased activity, a rapid heart rate, rapid breathing, an increase in apnea events, or feeding difficulties.

If the cause of anemia is not readily apparent, the NICU team may order diagnostic tests to look for evidence of bleeding or blood cell destruction. Babies with anemia of prematurity may undergo regular monitoring of their hemoglobin level and hematocrit to ensure they do not fall too low. A blood test called the *reticulocyte count* may be done intermittently to monitor how quickly the bone marrow is making new RBCs.

Treatment of Anemia of Prematurity

Babies without symptoms may not require any treatment. They may receive additional iron in their diet to ensure there is enough iron in their body to support RBC production once it begins. Some hospitals give regular injections of EPO to prevent or treat anemia of prematurity; however, this treatment remains controversial and is not routinely practiced in the United States. Babies with symptomatic anemia may require 1 or more RBC transfusions.

The likelihood of requiring a blood transfusion is related to the degree of prematurity at birth and the severity of illness. The more preterm a baby is, and the more significant the baby's health problems are, the greater the risk of requiring transfusions. There is no single rule for receiving a blood transfusion. Researchers continue to investigate the risks and benefits of different blood transfusion practices. Currently, more than half of babies born before 28 weeks' gestation will receive at least 1 blood transfusion.

> " Take some time at the beginning of the NICU experience and get organized. Appoint a willing friend to coordinate your other friends who want to help with groceries, meal prep, house cleaning, yard work, walking the dog, etc. This will help you maintain your sanity and your energy. "
>
> *Lisa, mother of **Frankie***

Problems Affecting the Preterm Baby's Heart

Patent Ductus Arteriosus (PDA)

While in the uterus, all healthy fetuses have a bridging artery that connects the 2 large blood vessels leaving the heart. This bridging artery is called the *ductus arteriosus.* Within a few days after a healthy term birth, the ductus arteriosus should close when the muscle surrounding the artery squeezes tightly. In preterm babies, the ductus arteriosus may remain open after birth or reopen in the weeks following birth. This is referred to as a *patent* (open) *ductus arteriosus* or *PDA.*

If the ductus arteriosus remains open, it may allow too much blood to enter the lungs and lead to heart and breathing problems. A PDA affects nearly half of babies born at less than 30 weeks' gestation or weighing less than 1,000 g (about 2 lb 3 oz). The more preterm a baby is at birth, the greater the risk of developing a PDA that causes trouble. The signs of a PDA often become apparent toward the end of the first week after birth and can, in some instances, continue for weeks or months.

Signs of a PDA

The signs of a PDA depend on how widely open the ductus arteriosus is, how much blood is flowing through it, and the direction in which the blood is flowing. Babies with a PDA

may have no problems. Some babies with a PDA may develop a *heart murmur,* breathing problems, an enlarged heart, feeding difficulties, or decreased urine output.

A heart murmur is a swooshing sound heard with a stethoscope. Heart murmurs are common in newborns, sometimes come and go, and do not necessarily indicate a problem. Sometimes, large PDAs have very soft murmurs or none at all, and very small PDAs have loud

Listening with a stethoscope gives the nurse information about **Lucy's** heart and lungs.

murmurs. The signs of a PDA may vary over the course of several hours and days.

Diagnosis of a PDA

If the NICU team suspects a PDA, an *echocardiogram* (*echo* for short) may be ordered. An echocardiogram is an ultrasound examination of the heart that can show if the ductus arteriosus is open, the direction of blood flow, and any signs that the heart is working too hard. Echocardiograms use sound waves to create moving images. There is no radiation exposure from an echocardiogram.

Treatment of a PDA

The treatment of a PDA depends on its size and the amount of difficulty it is causing your baby. A small PDA in an otherwise healthy preterm baby may cause few problems and may not need treatment. Many small preterm babies, however, do not tolerate a PDA and will need treatment.

If medical treatment is required, *indomethacin, acetaminophen,* or *ibuprofen* may be given. These medications are administered through an intravenous (IV) line or through a feeding tube and have similar functions. They interfere with a chemical in the body that relaxes the muscle surrounding the PDA. The goal is to make the muscle squeeze tightly, close the ductus, and, ultimately, cause it to "glue" shut. Some of the medications used to treat a PDA can affect kidney function. After receiving any of these medications, many babies will make less urine and retain water. This usually goes away in several days. Until it resolves, the NICU team may limit your baby's fluids and monitor kidney function using blood tests.

If the medication does not work or can't be used because of other problems, the PDA may be closed with a nonsurgical procedure in the cardiac catheterization laboratory (called *transcatheter PDA occlusion*) or through a surgical procedure (called a *ligation*).

Transcatheter PDA Closure

Some babies are eligible for PDA closure using a small occluding device. This device is inserted through a thin catheter by specialized cardiologists into a large vein in the groin and visualized with special x-rays before it is carefully placed into the PDA. The catheter is then removed, and a small bandage covers the catheter insertion site in the groin. The NICU team will periodically check the placement of the device with echocardiograms and x-rays.

Surgical Ligation for PDA Closure

Some infants are not candidates for a transcatheter PDA closure and will undergo a surgical PDA ligation. The procedure is performed by a cardiothoracic surgeon by making an incision between the ribs on the side of the baby's chest and closing the PDA with clips or stitches. When the surgery is over, there will be a bandage over the incision and possibly a chest tube to drain any bleeding. The chest tube is usually removed within a day or two after surgery. While recovering from surgery, some babies may be sicker for a few days than they were before surgery. During this time, they may temporarily have low blood pressure or more significant breathing problems.

Low Blood Pressure (Hypotension)

Blood pressure is controlled by several factors, including the tone of the tiny muscles that surround arteries, the amount of fluid inside your baby's blood vessels, and how hard your baby's heart is pumping blood. Babies have lower blood pressures than older children and adults. A healthy preterm baby has even lower normal blood pressures than a healthy full-term baby. Defining a healthy blood pressure for a preterm baby is difficult and depends on the baby's gestational age, age after birth, and health condition. Although it seems like a basic question, researchers are still trying to determine what a "normal" blood pressure is for a preterm baby and how low the blood pressure can be before treatment is needed.

In the NICU, blood pressure is measured using a tiny blood pressure cuff attached to an electronic machine. If the NICU team needs continuous monitoring of your baby's blood pressure, they may place an arterial line. An arterial line is a special catheter that is threaded into an artery and then attached to an electronic monitor. In the NICU, arterial lines are frequently placed into an artery in the wrist, ankle, or umbilical cord. If placed in the umbilical cord, the line is called an umbilical artery catheter (see Chapter 3).

Treatment of Low Blood Pressure

If treatment is needed, your baby's team will first try to identify the most likely cause of the low blood pressure.

Treatment Options for Low Blood Pressure in Preterm Babies

- Intravenous fluid or blood, called a volume *bolus,* to fill the blood vessels
- Intravenous medications that increase tone in the tiny muscles around arteries, increase the strength of heart contractions, and increase the heart rate. These medications are often called vasopressors (*pressors*) or inotropes.
- Intravenous steroids, such as *hydrocortisone.* This may be necessary when a baby's blood pressure remains very low despite receiving additional volume and other medications.

Problems Affecting the Preterm Baby's Intestines

The major organs of the gastrointestinal system are the stomach and intestines. The gastrointestinal system is responsible for processing food, absorbing nutrients, and removing waste by making baby's stool. Preterm babies are at risk of developing a serious intestinal problem called *necrotizing enterocolitis* (*NEC*).

Necrotizing Enterocolitis (NEC)

Necrotizing enterocolitis is a problem in which the cells lining the inside of the intestines become injured and swollen and may die. Damage to the bowel wall may be minor or quite serious. In severe cases, a hole may open in the intestinal wall, causing infection of the abdominal cavity and critical illness that can lead to death.

Risk Factors for NEC

Necrotizing enterocolitis is a disease that primarily affects preterm babies; however, some term babies may also get NEC. The more preterm a newborn is at birth, the greater the risk of developing NEC. In the United States, NEC occurs in 2% to 8% of babies born at less than 32 weeks' gestational age.

The reason that babies develop NEC is not completely understood, but NEC most often occurs after they have begun feedings. Preterm babies who receive only breast milk have a significantly lower risk of developing NEC.

Diagnosis of NEC

Babies with NEC may show a variety of signs, and the early signs may be very subtle. Other babies will have sudden changes in their belly (*abdomen*) and the signs will progress very quickly.

Early signs include abdominal swelling and difficulty digesting feedings. Babies with NEC may have blood in their stool or enlarged loops of bowel you can see by looking at their abdomen. There may be more general signs of illness, including less activity, more apnea, blotchy (*mottled*) skin, and abnormal body temperature.

The most common test for NEC is an abdominal x-ray. X-rays can identify bowel swelling and signs of gas in the bowel wall or liver. Bacteria invading the injured bowel wall may produce gas, which appears as little bubbles on the x-ray. This sign is called *pneumatosis intestinalis* and confirms the diagnosis of NEC.

Often, the x-ray shows mild problems but does not definitely diagnose NEC. In this case, the NICU team may obtain additional x-rays or an abdominal ultrasound. Caregivers may also obtain samples of blood, urine, and spinal fluid looking for signs of infection.

Treatment of NEC

Treatment depends on the baby's signs of illness. If the NICU team is not sure if the baby has NEC, feedings may be stopped and antibiotics given for 24 to 72 hours while additional tests are performed. When feedings are stopped, the caregivers may say the baby is NPO (Latin abbreviation for *nil per os),* which means no feedings are being given by mouth. If the signs of NEC go away and no evidence of NEC is found, feedings may be restarted and antibiotic treatment stopped. This is often called an *NEC evaluation* or *NEC workup.*

If the team thinks NEC is likely, your baby may have feedings stopped and antibiotics continued for a week or longer. A tube will be passed through your baby's nose or mouth and into the stomach (*nasogastric* or *orogastric tube*) to drain fluids and allow the intestines to rest. During this time, your baby will receive nutrition through an IV line.

Babies with NEC can be very ill and require close monitoring. X-rays may be obtained several times a day to check for rupture of the intestinal wall, which would show *free air* in the belly. Your baby may require oxygen or a ventilator for apnea. Additional fluids and medications may be needed for problems with low blood pressure, and your baby may need blood or platelet transfusions.

Most babies with NEC will improve with medications in 48 to 72 hours. Approximately one-quarter to one-half of babies with NEC will become sicker during the first 24 to 48 hours despite receiving medications and will require surgery.

Possible Complications of NEC

Rupture of the intestinal wall (*perforation*) is a serious complication of NEC that requires emergency surgery. Surgeons may place a small tube, called a *peritoneal drain,* in the abdomen to allow fluid and pus to drain out. Other babies may need a bigger surgery to open the belly (*laparotomy*) and remove parts of the sick intestine. However, after surgery, their condition may become very unstable and they get sicker. Despite antibiotic treatment and surgery, some babies will not get better and will die.

Your baby may come back from surgery with a temporary *ostomy* in place. An ostomy is a surgical opening on the surface of the baby's abdomen where the bowel has been attached so it can drain and have more time to heal. Stool drains from the ostomy opening into a collecting bag. In some patients, the ostomy can be removed (*taken down*) during another surgical procedure that reconnects the bowel, allowing for stool to again pass through the rectum. When possible, this surgery takes place weeks to months after the initial surgery.

Babies with severe NEC may need to have a lot of their intestine removed. The amount of healthy intestine left after surgery may be quite short and unable to absorb enough nutrients and water from the baby's food. This is called *short bowel syndrome* or *short gut syndrome.* Babies with short gut require prolonged IV nutrition and may need special formula and nutrient supplements.

Several weeks after healing, the bowel wall that was sick may develop scars that narrow the size of the bowel opening. Narrowing of the bowel is called a *stricture.* Babies with strictures have difficulty tolerating their feedings. Their abdomen may become bloated again and they may pass blood in their stool. These complications may require surgery to remove the scarred and narrow bowel.

Problems Affecting the Preterm Baby's Brain

The brain and nervous system begin developing during the third week of pregnancy, and development continues well beyond age 2 years. The brain uses a significant amount of energy and needs a constant supply of blood, nutrition, and oxygen. Because the brain is so complex and is still developing at the time of preterm birth, it is at risk of injury from many different causes.

Bleeding in the Brain (Hemorrhage)

New brain cells grow in an area deep within the brain called the *germinal matrix.* The germinal matrix sits next to a fluid-filled area of the brain called the *ventricles.* Blood vessels in this area carry a large amount of blood and are very fragile. During the hours to days before and after preterm birth, changes in blood flow may cause these vessels to break and bleed. The medical term for bleeding is *hemorrhage*. When bleeding occurs, the blood initially collects in the germinal matrix and may also fill the ventricles. The NICU team may call this a *germinal matrix hemorrhage*, an *intraventricular hemorrhage*, or *IVH*.

Risk Factors for Intraventricular Hemorrhage (IVH)

The greatest risk of bleeding in the brain occurs on the day of birth, and nearly all bleeding (75%) occurs during the first 3 days after birth. If a preterm baby has not had an IVH by the end of the first week, it is much less likely to occur.

The risk of IVH is directly related to the degree of prematurity and birth weight. Smaller and more preterm babies have a higher risk of bleeding and of the more severe types of bleeding. The brain's germinal matrix matures between 32 and 36 weeks' gestation. Following the maturation of the germinal matrix, the risk of this type of bleeding significantly decreases.

Symptoms of IVH

Frequently, there are no signs of a developing IVH. However, if the IVH is large, the baby may have a sudden change in condition, with low blood pressure, seizures, apnea, bradycardia, worsening anemia, and a bulging soft spot on the top of the head (*fontanel*).

Diagnosis of IVH

Hemorrhages are diagnosed using an ultrasound scan of the brain. Many NICUs routinely perform an ultrasound during a very preterm baby's first or second week after birth, even if there are no signs of hemorrhage. The ultrasound scanner is placed on the baby's scalp, over the soft spot, and sound waves are used to create images of the brain. Ultrasound is safe and does not expose the baby to any radiation.

If there is bleeding, it will be assigned a grade from 1 to 4 based on the amount of bleeding, its location, and the presence of enlargement or *dilation* of the ventricles. The smallest and most localized type of bleeding is assigned grade 1. More significant bleeds are assigned a higher number. A grade 4 bleed means there is bleeding into the substance of the brain, separate from the germinal matrix and ventricle. If bleeding is present, its progress and the reabsorption of blood will be monitored with ultrasound scans.

> ## Grading Brain Hemorrhages in Preterm Babies
>
> - **Grade 1** is the smallest amount of bleeding. Blood is only in the germinal matrix.
> - **Grade 2** means the bleeding has spread into the nearby ventricle.
> - **Grade 3** means the blood has entered the ventricles and is enlarging the ventricle.
> - **Grade 4** (also called an *intraparenchymal hemorrhage*) means there is bleeding into the substance of the brain, separate from the germinal matrix and ventricle. Often, babies with this type of bleeding also have a large intraventricular hemorrhage.

Complications of IVHs

Most hemorrhages are mild to moderate (grade 1 to 2), and nearly all of these will resolve with few short-term problems. A small percentage of newborns, fewer than 1 in 10, with mild or moderate hemorrhages may develop a blockage of fluid in their brains that causes swelling of the ventricles. This is called *hydrocephalus* or "water on the brain." Some babies with mild or moderate hemorrhages will go on to develop long-term developmental problems, such as cerebral palsy or learning disabilities. *Cerebral palsy* (CP) is a group of movement disorders that can affect a person's ability to move and maintain balance and posture. Signs of cerebral palsy often are first seen in early childhood.

Severe hemorrhages are more likely to result in short- and long-term problems. More than half of babies with grade 3 or 4 hemorrhages will develop hydrocephalus and long-term developmental problems, such as cerebral palsy, hearing loss, vision loss, and learning disabilities.

Hydrocephalus

Spinal fluid surrounds your baby's brain and spinal cord. *Hydrocephalus* occurs when the flow of spinal fluid is blocked or cannot be absorbed as it should. Following an IVH, blood in the spinal fluid may block the drainage system or scar the membranes that absorb it. The spinal fluid backs up in the ventricles, causing them to expand and push on the surrounding brain tissue. Although mild hydrocephalus may resolve by itself, it often requires an operation in which a neurosurgeon places a tube (a *reservoir* or a *shunt*) that drains the excess fluid.

Periventricular Leukomalacia

Periventricular leukomalacia (PVL) is abnormal development of the white part of the brain near the ventricles. The white part of the brain carries electrical messages between the brain and spinal cord. Periventricular leukomalacia may be detected by ultrasound scan or magnetic resonance imaging and looks like bright spots or small holes in the brain tissue. Even though the injury that caused PVL may have occurred before or shortly after birth, PVL may not be visible by ultrasound for several weeks after birth. Babies with PVL have a high risk of developing cerebral palsy.

Problems Affecting the Preterm Baby's Eyes

Your baby's eyes begin to develop during the first month of pregnancy, but the development is not complete until after birth.

Retinopathy of Prematurity (ROP)

The *retina* lines the inside of the eye and is a delicate light-sensitive membrane connected by the optic nerve to the brain. The retina begins developing around 16 weeks of gestation. It starts at the back of the eye and gradually spreads along the inside of the eyeball. The retina is made of living cells and needs a network of blood vessels to develop along with it. This development continues until close to a baby's due date. *Retinopathy of prematurity* (*ROP*) is a disease that occurs when abnormal blood vessels grow and spread throughout the developing retina.

Shortly after preterm birth, the normal growth of the retina and its blood vessels temporarily stops. We do not fully understand why this happens, but one factor is the rapid change in the amount of oxygen in the baby's blood after birth. Fetuses receive much less oxygen than babies need after birth.

After several weeks, the preterm baby's retina and blood vessels begin to grow again, but the blood vessels may not grow normally. There may be rapid, irregular growth of new blood vessels. These abnormal blood vessels are fragile and can leak, scarring the retina and pulling it out of position. A retina that is pulled away from the back of the eye is called a *retinal detachment*. Retinal detachment is the main cause of severe visual impairment and blindness in ROP.

Risk Factors for ROP

The risk of ROP increases with decreasing gestational age and birth weight. Retinopathy of prematurity is usually seen in babies less than 30 weeks' gestational age. After that, the retinal vessels have developed enough that they are not at risk. More than half of babies delivered at less than 27 weeks' gestation will develop some ROP.

Higher levels of oxygen in the blood might play some role in the development of ROP. Consequently, the blood oxygen saturation in all preterm babies receiving oxygen is carefully monitored. The goal is to ensure that babies receive enough oxygen to support their body's needs while limiting excess oxygen that may contribute to ROP. Most NICUs use pulse oximetry to monitor oxygen saturation and have target levels that they hope to maintain while the baby is receiving supplemental oxygen. In real life, this can be very difficult to do, as babies often have fluctuating oxygen levels.

Still, ROP develops in some babies with lower oxygen levels and does not develop in others with higher oxygen levels. There have even been cases of ROP in babies who did not receive any additional oxygen. Because the cause of ROP is not fully understood, it is not possible to completely prevent this problem or accurately predict which babies will develop ROP.

Diagnosis of ROP

Babies born at less than 30 weeks' gestation or weighing less than 1,500 g (3 lb 5 oz) usually have their eyes examined by an eye specialist (*ophthalmologist*) when they are approximately 4 to 5 weeks old. Some babies weighing 1,500 to 2,000 g or delivered between 30 and 32 weeks' gestation will be examined if their medical provider thinks they are at risk. In some institutions, photographs of the retina are taken with a special camera and electronically sent to an ophthalmologist for evaluation.

Before the eye examination, drops will be placed in the baby's eyes to enlarge (*dilate*) the pupils so the retina can be viewed. The ophthalmologist uses a special lens to look into the eyes and evaluate the progress of retinal development. The ophthalmologist may simply say the retina is still immature. This means no ROP was seen; however, the retina and its blood vessels are still developing and are at risk of ROP. The ophthalmologist will perform repeat eye examinations until the retina is mature.

If abnormal blood vessels are seen, the ophthalmologist will describe the ROP according to a standard system. This includes a number that describes the severity of the condition (*stage*) and a description of which portion of the retina is involved (*zone*). The term *PLUS disease* is used if the ophthalmologist sees very aggressive ROP with thick and twisted blood vessels. Retinopathy of prematurity may involve 1 or both eyes. Depending on the maturity of the retina and presence of ROP, the ophthalmologist will schedule additional follow-up examinations.

 In the NICU, it was 5 steps forward and 3 steps backward.

*Parina, mother of **Isaac** and **Eliza***

Treatment of ROP

In mild cases, ROP resolves by itself and leaves no permanent damage. Babies with more severe ROP can develop poor vision or even blindness and may require injection of a medication or laser surgery.

Injection of a medication directly into the eye that blocks the chemical signal to grow new blood vessels (*anti-VEGF therapy*) is one treatment option for severe ROP. Ophthalmologists have been using these injections for many years. Several medications are being studied for treatment of ROP, but all work in a similar way. By temporarily blocking the signal for new blood vessel growth, these medications can reverse or slow the progression of ROP. Frequently, ROP will return several weeks after the injection, and treated babies may still require laser surgery. However, by delaying the need for laser surgery, the baby's retina may have more time to mature and require less laser treatment.

With laser surgery, a laser beam carefully directed through the baby's pupil and into the eye destroys the outer areas of the retina, slowing or reversing the abnormal vessel growth. The baby may lose some vision to the side (*peripheral vision*), but the goal of laser surgery is to prevent retinal detachments and save the baby's ability to see straight ahead.

Babies with the most advanced ROP who develop a retinal detachment may need additional surgery.

Problems Affecting the Preterm Baby's Skin

Intact skin is an important barrier. It protects the body from invading bacteria, helps maintain fluid balance by preventing excess water loss, and provides insulation, preventing heat loss. Preterm skin is a less effective barrier and more prone to injury than fully mature skin.

The Preterm Baby's Skin

You may notice that a very preterm baby's skin initially appears shiny, sticky, and gelatinous with visible veins. More mature babies have a dry, flaky layer of skin. After birth, preterm skin matures quickly. You will notice your baby's skin becoming dry and flaky. This is a normal and healthy change. Within a few weeks, a preterm baby's skin is similar to the skin of a term baby.

Heat Loss

At birth, a newborn moves from the warm uterine environment to the cooler delivery room. For the first time, newborns must control their own temperature. As far back as the early 1900s, researchers found that carefully maintaining a normal body temperature improved survival of preterm newborns. If preterm newborns use energy for heat production, they may use up their energy stores, develop low blood sugar, and stop growing.

Preterm babies like **Jack,** who are less than 32 weeks' gestation, are covered in plastic wrap or placed inside a polyethylene plastic bag to prevent heat loss at birth.

Maintaining a normal body temperature is a major focus of care from the moment of birth. In the delivery room, your baby will be placed under a radiant warmer. Right after birth, babies less than about 32 weeks' gestation may be covered up to their neck with a clear plastic sheet or bag similar to the plastic wrap/bag you use in your kitchen. Shortly after birth, preterm newborns may be moved to an incubator. The incubator keeps your baby warm by controlling the environmental temperature and blocking cool air currents that could move across the body. Very preterm newborns may also have humidity added to the air in the incubator to prevent water loss from the baby's skin.

Special Care for Preterm Skin

All preterm babies receive special skin care. Skin care includes gentle handling; avoidance of lotions, ointments, or other substances (unless medically indicated); use of special tape that is gentle to the skin; avoidance of adhesives; and use of special transparent wound dressings. These clear adhesive dressings can be used over skin irritations to promote healing or over places where IV lines or catheters have been inserted to protect these sites and reduce the risk of infection. A soft, easy-to-remove barrier may be placed between the tape and the newborn's skin.

Even with careful attention to skin care, some preterm newborns may develop areas of skin irritation. Preventing irritation and skin breakdown is an important but challenging goal for neonatal care providers. New research is constantly changing neonatal skin care practices, and each NICU may have its own skin care protocol.

Knowledge Is Power

This chapter has described many common problems that can occur in preterm babies. The wide range of potential problems may seem overwhelming. It is important to remember that being at risk for a problem does not mean a baby will definitely develop it. Many preterm babies will experience one of the problems described in this chapter; some will experience several; and, unfortunately, a few will experience many. Knowledge of your baby's risks for specific problems enables you and your NICU team to monitor your baby carefully, identify signs of developing problems, and begin treatment quickly. Your team can provide more specific information about your baby's risks based on gestational age, birth weight, and unique health conditions.

Alexander

(Alex)

Born at 26 weeks
· · · · · · · · · · · · · ·

My first pregnancy was very healthy and fairly easy. I gave birth naturally, at 37 weeks and 6 days. My second pregnancy seemed to be going as smoothly as my first; however, I was a little more tired. Growing a baby while keeping up with an infant at home was a lot!

I was 26 weeks pregnant with our second son when things took an unexpected turn. It was my day off, so I went to my prenatal Pilates session, got a facial, and did some gro-

cery shopping. When I got home, I suddenly felt dizzy, so I grabbed some crackers and sat down. Seconds later, I rushed to the bathroom and discovered I was bleeding. At that moment, I knew something was wrong.

I called my husband Anthony and he was on his way home. I then called my OB-GYN who told me to go to OB triage where she would meet me. When Anthony arrived, he started packing our hospital bags and I chuckled. I said, "We are not having the baby today! It is way too early! They'll stop this."

Minutes later as we rushed to the hospital, I braced myself as my contractions started. By the time we arrived at the hospital, I was bleeding profusely. A sonogram was done to make sure the baby was safe and he was, but his feet were down and he was just dancing around in my belly. I asked my OB what

After a cesarean birth, Alex is stable with a CPAP mask in place and briefly visits his mother before going to the NICU.

could be done to stop the contractions and her answer caught me off guard. I was fully dilated, she told me, and there was no stopping this baby. Our world was completely rocked.

I was prepped for an emergency C-section and within minutes our mighty Alexander was born at just 26 weeks' gestation, weighing only 1 pound 15 ounces. Alexander was quickly rolled off to the NICU where he would spend the next 126 days.

Less than 36 hours after Alexander was born, we nearly lost him. My husband Anthony was at Alexander's bedside and witnessed Alexander's oxygen saturation levels drop. Anthony ran up to the postpartum floor and rushed me back to the NICU in a wheelchair. When we arrived, Alexander's room was filled with the NICU team trying

During his NICU stay, Alex required various levels of respiratory support. In this photo, Alex is on CPAP.

Alex's family visits him in the NICU.

to save him, and thankfully they did. As a result of the drop in oxygen levels, imaging of his brain showed a grade 3 and grade 4 brain hemorrhage.

We were now 2 days into our NICU journey and we quickly put a routine into place. We spent our mornings at home with AJ before dropping him off at childcare, then we headed to the NICU for 8 to 9 hours. Anthony and I spent hours at Alex's beside. We made it a point to be there for all rounds with the neonatologist and specialists and for other testing. We would both go home to have dinner and bedtime with AJ, then one of us would return to the NICU to do a bedtime routine of stories and prayers with Alex. Some nights we would have a hard time leaving his side and would fall asleep at the hospital.

During his time in the NICU, he had various levels of breathing support via the oscillator, ventilator, SiPap, bubble CPAP and high-pressure nasal cannula. He also had heart surgery for a PDA ligation at just 2 weeks old. Just a few minutes before the surgery, the NICU team allowed big brother AJ in to meet his baby brother for the first time. Our priest was also welcomed in as he baptized and confirmed Alex into our Catholic faith prior to the procedure.

Our NICU journey was quite the rollercoaster as we celebrated all the littlest milestones while also experiencing setbacks including bradycardia and desaturation episodes, liver difficulties, bone density issues, ROP concerns, gut difficulties, feeding challenges, and so much more.

After 3 months in the NICU, Alexander was breathing on his own and we just needed to get him to eat by mouth. I was breast-feeding for a short time, but it became more stressful than anything. Due to reflux and excessive spit-ups, he was not gaining enough weight so my breast milk needed to be fortified. Shortly after fortifying, more weight gain issues continued along with concerns about his bone density, so my breast milk was further supplemented with high-calorie formula. After quite some time, Alex was moved to a 30-calorie formula and at that point I felt defeated. But I wanted to provide what was best for him, which was the high-calorie formula for all his feeds.

As discussions of discharge began, we were told that several tests and items on a checklist needed to be done. This included another brain MRI to follow up on the damage that occurred when he was 2 days old. The MRI of his brain confirmed severe damage, but his future was unknown and we already knew we were ready to give him the best possible life.

After 126 long days, we got to welcome Alex home. Fast forward to today, Alex is 3 years old and eats anything and everything by mouth. He has gone through intensive physical therapy and occupational therapy since discharge. He is walking with an irregular gait, but he is fully walking, climbing, running, and keeping up with his 2 brothers and his friends.

Alex, his parents, and his big brother enjoy family time at home.

He still sees several specialists for his diagnoses that include cerebral palsy and spastic diplegia. He wears braces to help stretch his legs, he receives physical and occupational therapy and chiropractic adjustments to help him move forward with his gross motor skills, fine motor skills, and behavior.

He is thriving. He is a happy, intelligent, outgoing, and wild 3-year-old who loves his big and little brothers so much.

Stacy and Anthony, parents of Alexander

Alex develops physical and social skills when he plays on the swing in the yard.

Ellie

Born at 39 weeks

No one ever expects to have a baby in the NICU. When you get pregnant, you dream of having the perfect delivery, the perfect newborn phase, and all the beauty that comes from a brand-new baby. I had the easiest pregnancy out of all 3 of my pregnancies. It was such a dream. My third baby, Ellie Faith, was to be my last baby. I knew going into pregnancy that I would savor every moment.

I was scheduled to be induced at 39 weeks and 1 day. My middle child's labor was only one hour long, and my doctor wanted to have a controlled environment so she wouldn't be born in the car. On the morning of my scheduled induction, my water broke. We got in the car and made it to the hospital. It was an amazing labor and delivery, and out of all 3 children the easiest. At 9:02 am my sweet Ellie Faith was born. The amazing nurses laid her on my chest and I was able to look into her eyes. I remember thinking how wonderful it was to see her.

At 9:20 am, I noticed her head was rocking back and forth as she tried to breathe. It sounded like a tapping noise. It seemed as if every breath was a struggle. I didn't think much of it and the nurse asked if we wanted a family picture.

After the pictures were taken, the nurse noticed her breathing was getting worse. She went from a normal new baby color to a blue/gray color. The nurse scooped her up. That would be the last time I'd hold her on her birthday. A frenzy of activity followed. The nurses called in a pediatrician to help and I heard, "I can't get a pulse ox over 40%." I looked at Matt, completely blindsided and terrified.

Ellie is on ECMO. She has had 2 tubes (cannulas) surgically placed into large blood vessels in her neck (visible on the lower left). Her support includes an endotracheal tube, umbilical catheters, and numerous intravenous lines.

We waited for about an hour and then 4 nurses, a doctor, and a medical student walked in. I immediately thought Ellie had died and they were bringing people to comfort us. The doctor started with, "We had to intubate her because her heart rate got down into the 60s." I did not hear anything after that. I immediately started to sob. How is it a perfect pregnancy and delivery could end up like this? My whole body went numb and it felt like a bad dream.

They brought me a wheelchair and took Matt and me down the hall to the NICU. As the door opened, I lost it again. There she was, completely blue and lifeless. Eyes closed, hands cold and motionless, mouth forced open by the plastic tubing down her throat, leads all

over her chest, tape across her face and body keeping everything in place, machines and tubes surrounding and running in and out of her tiny plastic box. Her pulse ox was down into the 60% range and there were alarms going off. She looked like an experiment out of a sci-fi movie and it was almost too overwhelming for me. How was this the same perfect baby I had just delivered 2 hours ago whose blue eyes opened up so perfectly and looked into mine? I placed my hand on her and tried to imagine she was just like my other 2 children but couldn't get past the situation in front of me. My heart was breaking.

Ellie's parents visit the NICU for the first time. Melissa is supported by a person in front, who holds her arm, and by her husband who stands behind her. The nurse at the warmer helps Melissa touch her baby.

The neonatologist then explained to us that the university children's hospital was sending a helicopter to come get her. That is when I knew this would be a long uphill climb. The cardiologist said she may need ECMO to allow her heart and lungs to rest and heal. My husband Matt, looking for a straightforward, authentic, and real bottom-line opinion, asked the neonatologist how sick he really thought she was. The doctor said, "This is the second sickest baby I've seen this year." That made us take a breath. I remember thinking, *is this how it will end? Right after I just met her? How do I tell Emma that her baby sister died?* Emma had been so excited. She and I would talk all the time about what it would be like to play with a sister, share a room, play with dolls, dress up, and be best friends for life. How do you even begin to process this?

Ellie, after she had started to improve and ECMO was removed.

Ellie, 9 days old, snuggles with her mother.

We returned to our room to debrief. I told Matt that we needed everyone we knew to begin to pray for Ellie as soon as possible. So he took to Facebook and posted our first update. Pretty soon prayers began to rise from every corner of the globe. We truly felt a peace and grace enter our room.

A few hours later, my doctor approved a special early discharge and, finally, we arrived at the children's hospital. I could not believe Ellie was in an ICU. I was still in a state of shock. There were about 5 nurses in her room setting up machines, adjusting cords, and getting her settled. It was surreal, in a nightmare sort of way. I tried to bond with her, but it was nearly impossible to not focus on everthing happening around her. This was not the birthday that I had imagined for Ellie. Not only was I completely blindsided by what happened, but no one could tell me why it happened.

The next 4 hours were the longest of our lives. We sat in a sterile white room with nothing but 2 chairs and a box of tissues. We rode the waves of faith, uncertainty, and despair. In those moments, your mind plays tricks on you—taking you from dreaming about miraculous healing to making funeral arrangements.

The doctor entered at about 2 am and said, "It took a lot longer than expected, but she was successfully placed on ECMO. We are not sure if she will last through the night." Twenty-four hours after my water broke, we finally had our first piece of good news.

The next morning, we woke up devastated, but not defeated. We walked into her room and noticed they had added a bunch of wires to her head. The nurse explained that she had 14 seizures after going on ECMO and that the EEG monitor would pick them up if she had more. The possibility of long-term brain damage was something new to think about. Would she be brain-dead or mentally disabled? Would we ever get to take her home? These questions were swirling in my head.

Each morning, the doctors and nurses would go room by room talking through each case and the plan/goals for the day. We quickly found their meetings were filled with lots of useful information, including what they were planning on doing with Ellie for the day, new information about what they thought happened, and anything else pertinent for the day or week. Matt took meticulous notes. They had diagnosed her with PPHN (persistent pulmonary hypertension of the newborn) and HIE (hypoxic ischemic encephalopathy), but they couldn't tell me *why* it happened. They said it was a fluke.

After that first day, her healing was nothing short of *miraculous*!

25 days after her birth we went home with our beautiful baby girl.

Ellie was diagnosed with brain damage in her thalamus and the frontal parietal lobe of her brain from the extreme lack of oxygen and has been in physical, occupational, and speech therapy 3 times a week since she was born. She is about 6 months cognitively and physically behind, but the doctors honestly cannot believe that she is doing as well as she is. She stuns every single medical professional she meets.

Even though the NICU was an incredibly hard place to be, we experienced the darkest and brightest aspects of human life. It's been like watching every sermon, verse, devotional, and word on faith and healing happen in real time. It's a beautiful thing to say that you've witnessed and experienced those things. Ellie continues to be a light to everyone who meets her. She is a complete miracle and has changed many lives already.

Melissa, mother of Ellie

Ellie, 5 years old.

Frankie

Born at 29 weeks

I was admitted to the hospital after a prenatal appointment at 27 weeks' gestation. We actually were told at that appointment that I might be delivering Frankie that evening and from the moment we heard that, we were pretty terrified. I was put on bed rest, diagnosed with preeclampsia. Frankie was delivered via emergency C-section 2 weeks later.

Frankie, at birth.

We knew it would be an emergency C-section. The labor and delivery staff made sure that I understood what that was going to look like. They prepared me with everything I needed to know. It was quick and I was able to see Frankie minutes later. They wheeled my bed in to see her as the nurses and doctors were evaluating and connecting Frankie to all her monitors. Frankie was 1 pound 11 ounces and 14¼ inches long.

I honestly believe I was in complete shock. Everything they told me, I never processed. I know this because my husband recorded many of our conversations with staff, and I don't remember any of it.

Physical exhaustion, mental exhaustion, intravenous magnesium, and now your child is born and you need to produce milk and pump every 3 hours … it's incredibly exhausting. So, ironically, Frankie entered the world during the opening ceremony of the summer Olympics and we were having our own opening ceremony—life of preemie parents in the NICU.

She was born and still is a thriver! While I teach, she learns at an in-home child care 5 days a week. I would have never thought she would be in a child care with GERMS! She counts to 50, spells her name, rides a bike with training wheels, takes ballet, can brush her own teeth, is potty trained (wow, that was so easy compared to other things), uses technology quite well, loves books, loves the outdoors, and, yes, throws little tantrums!

Frankie, at age 3.

It's awesome to see her growth and development with eating and sleeping. Those things were our concern and she has made such fantastic progress. I would have never imagined her cutting her own food, enjoying so many different types of food, but, most importantly, she eats with no pain or aversions.

I rarely refer to her as a preemie. She was born a preemie, but she is all toddler now. She is 3½ years old! I will never forget our time spent in the hospital and the challenges we faced for several years. These babies thrive. They can thrive and they do thrive. **Read more about Frankie in "Where Are They Now?" in the appendix.**

Lisa, mother of Frankie

CHAPTER 6

Parenting in the NICU

> " We knew it was going to be a
> long journey. We knew that we were
> going on a roller coaster ride, and we
> needed to hold on tight! We knew that
> we literally had to take it hour by hour,
> day by day, week by week, and
> month by month.
>
> *Sophany and Mike, parents of **Eliana***
>
> "

You are an important part of your baby's life in the neonatal intensive care unit (NICU) and a valuable member of your baby's health care team. At first, you may feel nervous around the equipment and NICU staff, but you have a bond with your baby that no other member of the NICU team can match. You will learn how to care for your baby in a context of love that will continue long after the NICU stay is behind you.

Parenting in the NICU often poses many challenges, but you can meet them. A positive experience depends on forming a working partnership with the NICU team and getting involved in your baby's care. This helps you learn about your baby, grow as a parent, and prepare for your baby's homecoming.

Forming a Partnership With the NICU Team

Getting to know the daily NICU routine and providing care for your baby helps break down some of the challenges in NICU parenting. Open and honest communication with the health care team creates trusting partnerships. You are an essential member of your baby's team and your input and involvement are important in preparing and carrying out your baby's plan of care. In a successful partnership, planning for your baby's discharge begins early in the NICU stay.

Ask Questions and Learn as You Go

No question is silly or unnecessary. Take as much time as you need to discuss your concerns and ask questions. Don't be afraid to say that you just don't understand something or need the

information presented in a different way. People learn in various ways and at different paces. The NICU team expects you to have plenty of questions.

Forgetting what you've been told also is normal when you're distracted by the NICU environment. Don't be embarrassed or afraid to ask for the information again.

Colson was born with an abdominal defect and underdeveloped lungs.

> " Colson remained in the NICU for 7 months. The NICU staff was very supportive and informative and they valued our opinions as parents when making medical decisions regarding Colson's health. "
>
> *Jewel, mother of **Colson***

Write Down Questions as You Think of Them

Although families often have many questions about their baby, when they get the chance to ask them, no one can remember the questions. To avoid this problem, write down your questions as they occur to you. Keep the list in your purse or wallet, make a reminder on your phone, or start a folder on your tablet so you'll have your questions ready when you need them. You can use the same system to write down the answers to your questions and file them for future reference.

Communication Starters

Starting your questions or ideas with conversation openers can help you reach your goals. These openers allow you to give and receive information at the same time.

- "Would you think about …?"
- "I read about … Do you think that might work?"
- "Can you share with me the pros and cons of …?"
- "I'm not familiar with … Can you tell me more?"
- "What if we tried …?"

Questions That Don't Have a Clear Answer

It is important to feel comfortable and satisfied with the answers to your questions. Keep in mind, however, that you may not always get the answer you want. Some questions have no clear answers. In other cases, too many variables exist to permit a specific answer. Lack of a conclusive answer can be frustrating. Acknowledging your frustration to your baby's team may be helpful. Chances are that team members are also frustrated when they cannot give you a conclusive answer.

> I am a transgender man and I gave birth to my baby. This NICU respected that I am Pascal's dad, not his mom. For trans or LGB (lesbian, gay, or bisexual) parents who land in the NICU, ask for your pronouns and title to be respected. Post a note for staff near your baby so you don't have to explain over and over. Not worrying about how I would be referred to meant I could focus on him, instead of building a protective wall around that part of my being.

*Alex, father of **Pascal***

Challenges of Parenting

Learning how to touch and hold your baby and read your baby's cues is an important part of parenting. However, NICU parents may feel that obstacles stand between them and their baby. Parenting will get more comfortable as you learn more about your baby and as your baby starts to mature and feel better. In the meantime, it helps to know about common parenting barriers and how to deal with them.

Separation

If your baby is in a NICU some distance from your home, family members may be separated from one another. It may be difficult to find an affordable place to stay near your baby. Low-cost temporary housing is sometimes available for parents. Some hospitals may make rooms available or have arrangements with nearby hotels for parents and family. Ask about these resources and use them when you are able.

If you are parenting from a long distance, set up a phone call schedule and communicate often with your baby's health care team. Strategies to help you cope with long-distance parenting may include joining rounds by phone, using online video systems, or receiving emails and photos to update you on your baby's progress and involve you in your baby's daily activities. Try not to feel guilty if you are not able to be there as much as you would like. Keep in touch with your baby's NICU team—they know you care. For parents at a distance, the chance to room-in (see Chapter 8) before discharge is valuable. Ask the team about the possibilities.

> ❝ Anthony and I spent hours at Alex's bedside. We made it a point to be there for all rounds with the neonatologist and specialists and for other testing. We would both go home to have dinner and bedtime with AJ, then one of us would return to the NICU to do a bedtime routine of stories and prayers with Alex. Some nights we would have a hard time leaving his side and we would fall asleep at the hospital. ❞
>
> *Stacy and Anthony, parents of **Alex***

Exhaustion

Many parents find the overall atmosphere of the NICU stressful and exhausting. Rest is essential for both parents, but for the birthing parent, it's especially important for recovering after childbirth and for milk production. Many NICUs have a parent lounge where you can go when you are tired or overwhelmed. Your NICU team will tell you where you can rest, recharge digital devices, eat, and use the bathroom.

Devices and Equipment

Many mechanical barriers come between you and your baby in the NICU. Your baby's incubator can be intimidating at first. You may hesitate to break through this barrier and touch your baby. Tubing and monitor wires can tangle like vines in the jungle, and you don't want to risk pulling something loose. All of this can make caring for your baby a challenge, but the NICU team can help you work around these obstacles.

Shana takes a moment to rest her head against **Abel's** incubator. Recovering from a complicated birth and caring for your NICU baby can be exhausting.

Bedside equipment, such as this wall of pumps and monitors, can be an intimidating obstacle for parents in the NICU.

Abel's nurse helps his mother manage his endotracheal tube, wires, and cables so that she can hold him in both hands.

> 66 Don't be afraid to be as involved as early as possible. The more you help, the faster you become comfortable, and it is so rewarding. 99

*Mary Ellen, mother of **Meridith***

Psychological Barriers

Parents report a range of emotions about the NICU environment. How you feel may depend on whether you were expecting your baby to need NICU care, your baby's condition, your own condition, and if you have had any previous NICU experience. At first, the NICU may seem like a foreign land. You may feel uncertain and wonder about any unspoken "rules" or expectations. You may fear that if you ask too many questions or become demanding, you will annoy the staff, and your baby may not receive good care. These fears are normal but unfounded. They will lessen as you become more familiar and involved with the staff and the NICU routine. If your baby's birth didn't happen as you planned, you and your partner may also mourn the loss of that planned experience. You may have written a detailed birth plan about how you wanted your labor and delivery to unfold. Unfortunately, your preterm or complicated birth may not have met many of these expectations. Developing a new set of goals for making progress is an important part of NICU parenthood. These new goals may include weaning off of a ventilator, holding your baby, or breastfeeding for the first time.

> " After our first week in the NICU, my husband returned to work to save his time off for when we were discharged. He would come and visit us before and after work, then go home to take care of the pets and house. That was a good decision for us. "
>
> *Mary Ellen, mother of **Meridith***

Guilt and Anger

For nearly all parents, the NICU is a new and stressful place. Many parents feel guilty after the birth of a baby who needs care in a NICU. You may ask yourself and the NICU team, "What did I do to cause this?" or "What could I have done to prevent this?" Parents reflect on their lives since the day they learned about the pregnancy, wondering if they could have changed the outcome.

You may feel powerless and angry that your birth experience did not go as expected. You might find yourself angry at your family and friends or even your partner. ("They just don't understand.") As uncomfortable as it may be, you may also feel angry at your baby. ("Why couldn't you have waited for just a few more weeks?")

It helps to know that most pregnancy and birth complications are not anyone's fault and many NICU admissions are unexpected. Still, many parents feel they may somehow have done something—or not done something—to make it happen. Share these feelings with your NICU team. Often, they can provide answers and reassurance.

Attachment

Some parents admit feeling jealous of nurses who do everything well and seem to meet their baby's needs better than they can. But as you spend time with your new baby, you will find yourself becoming the expert. Actively participating in your baby's care will help you feel more like a parent and resolve many of those feelings.

If your baby was very ill, you may also have a lingering fear that your baby could die. This may complicate feelings of love and attachment. Give yourself some time to sort out your feelings, and remember that loving feelings for your baby will grow stronger over time. You may find it helpful to discuss your feelings with your baby's doctor, nurse, social worker, or another support person.

> ❝ Another thing I have forgiven myself for, but didn't at the time, was my inability to love my son in the first few weeks. At 24 weeks' gestation, he didn't look like the babies you see in pictures or on social media. It was a defense mechanism, I think. I didn't have anyone in my social network who had delivered a baby so early, or even preterm at all. That was isolating. ❞
>
> *Robyn, mother of **Auggie***

The "Baby Blues" and Postpartum Depression

Pregnancy and childbirth bring about tremendous physical and emotional changes, with dramatic variation in hormone levels. These changes may affect brain function and can lead to depression. This is more common than many people realize, and many birthing parents experience the "baby blues" to some extent. Symptoms may begin in the early days after the baby's birth and include feeling anxious or irritable, with mood swings. Many birthing parents find themselves suddenly tearful, and there may be unwelcome changes in appetite or sleep patterns. The "baby blues" should subside within 2 weeks, but sometimes symptoms will begin later or extend beyond that time frame. These feelings usually go away on their own and typically do not last for more than 2 weeks.

Postpartum depression is a more serious concern and can occur anytime during the first year after childbirth. It is more common in birthing parents who experience additional stresses, such as those of parenting a baby with special care needs. Adoptive parents who have not actually birthed their babies may also find themselves struggling with this common condition. The parent who is experiencing this may not recognize their symptoms or may seek help without assistance from their partner or another support person. Your new baby needs parents to be at their best, so it is vitally important to seek expert help if symptoms last longer than 2 weeks.

Postpartum depression can occur in the non-birthing parent too. Research is now showing that up to 10% of non-birthing parents experience significant depression in the first year of their baby's life. The risk is higher if their baby is in the NICU and if their partner also has signs of depression. The non-birthing parent may feel overwhelmed, unprepared to parent, inadequate, exhausted, anxious, moody, or angry. They may withdraw from relationships, lose motivation to do things they previously enjoyed, and/or start working much more or much less. The non-birthing parent may notice changes in their mood or behavior, but not

Please use this QR code to go directly to www. healthychildren.org/ English/ages-stages/ prenatal/delivery-beyond/Pages/Dads-Can-Get-Postpartum-Depression-Too.aspx.

recognize these as signs of depression. Some may deny their symptoms because they think that postpartum depression only occurs in the birthing parent. While symptoms of anxiety and depression may appear several months before birth, the greatest risk of developing depression in non-birthing parents occurs when the baby is 3 to 6 months old. More information about depression in non-birth parents is available from the American Academy of Pediatrics at **www.healthychildren.org/English/ages-stages/prenatal/delivery-beyond/Pages/Dads-Can-Get-Postpartum-Depression-Too.aspx**.

Persistent symptoms that signal the need for professional intervention include feeling depressed and disinterested in activities that are usually enjoyable, having a hard time concentrating, and experiencing continued feelings of anxiety, guilt, unworthiness, or hopelessness. Some parents may become so troubled that they consider harming themselves or others. Whether symptoms are mild or severe, postpartum depression can be successfully managed. Talk with your physician or a member of your NICU team about obtaining professional assistance.

Some parents may become so troubled that they consider harming themselves or others. If you're having these feelings, please call the 988 Suicide & Crisis Lifeline. Call or text 988, or chat **988lifeline.org** to connect with mental health professionals in the United States who can support you during a mental health crisis. You may also call a neighbor, friend, or family member so that they can be with you while you call for help.

Whether symptoms are mild or severe, postpartum depression can be successfully managed. Talk with your physician or a member of your NICU team about obtaining professional assistance so that you can begin your recovery as soon as possible.

> " I think I was most surprised about the grief and pain from the trauma after almost losing our daughter. I thought after we left the NICU that emotionally I would be fine. It has taken me almost 3 years to come to grips with what happened in the NICU and there are times when I still feel the pain of the situation. "
>
> *Melissa, mother of **Ellie***

Your Partner, Your Family, Your Friends

Family Imbalance

This can be a highly stressful time for parents, marked by feelings of physical and emotional separation. Some couples offer each other remarkable support, growing closer and building

their bond through this experience. Others may feel separated by anger, guilt, denial, blame, or feelings of failure and uncertainty. Parents and other family members may be doing everything they can to cope with the situation and not have any energy left to support each other. Many parents say they don't tell each other what they are thinking or feeling. In these cases, stress and mis-understandings can multiply because everyone is too exhausted to sort things out. When issues are not discussed, marriages, partnerships, and family relationships can suffer.

Eliana's parents comfort their baby and each other on Eliana's birth day.

Partners May Cope Differently

After discharge from the hospital, NICU parents may get less sleep than they need and grab meals on the run. Some parents feel they have more jobs than their partner—and no time for themselves or the rest of their family. One parent may be making daily trips to the NICU and wonder why their partner does not seem more involved.

Some NICU parents cope by backing off, leaving their partner to assume most of the parenting role. They may busy themselves at work to restore a sense of normalcy and control in their lives. A parent who feels uncomfortable in the NICU may cope with their helplessness by avoiding the NICU.

If parents are feeling stressed but coping in very different ways, it is no wonder their relation-ship becomes strained. When you are in crisis, you may not have the energy to help others. It can be difficult to talk to one another and understand the other person's point of view.

Although open, expressive communication may be difficult, it is important to maintain your relationships. Seek help from other parents who have experienced the NICU, from your spiri-tual counselor, or from caring professionals. Many couples find they need emotional support and professional assistance to work through difficulties and keep their relationships strong.

It may be hard to take time out for yourself, as well as ask for help; however, taking time for yourself is important to restore the energy you need to deal with the NICU. As soon as you feel you are able, take a day off from the NICU, make a date with your partner, and meet your own personal needs. This time-out is essential for your well-being. Don't think of it as taking time away from your baby.

Drugs and alcohol may temporarily help you forget your problems, but they only complicate things in the long run. If you have a substance dependence disorder, you will likely be unable to face the realities of parenting without professional help. If your problems seem overwhelming, seek help from your family health care professional or ask your baby's social worker for help.

> **“** Take care of yourselves, take time to leave the room to take a walk, go have lunch, sleep in your own bed, whatever you need to do to make yourself feel better. You can't take care of your baby if you don't take care of yourself first. **”**
>
> *Mary Ellen, mother of **Meridith***

Getting acquainted with your baby takes time. This father is now comfortable enough with the NICU environment to enjoy skin-to-skin care with his baby.

Courtesy of University of Washington Medical Center, Seattle, WA.

What to Tell Your Other Children

If you have other children, they will want to know when the baby is coming home or where the baby is. Tell them as simply as you can about their sibling. Be honest, and try to answer your children's questions at their level. Remember that for younger children, a baby they cannot see is difficult to imagine. Showing them photos can help them see their new brother or sister as a real person.

It can be especially difficult for toddlers and preschoolers to understand what is happening. Young children may not understand why their routines are disrupted after the new baby's arrival and say things like, "I hate that baby." These feelings are normal. They also need to be reassured that the baby's illness is not their fault. Simple explanations and "exchanging" gifts with the baby help young children feel important and involved. Some NICUs have sibling support classes that you can attend with your toddlers or young children.

You will be understandably upset by the birth of a baby who needs intensive care, and even young children will know something is wrong. If you leave your children out of this experience

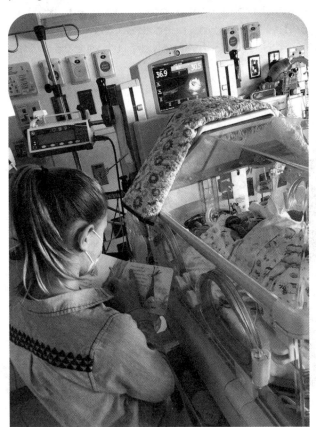

or neglect to discuss everyone's feelings, they are likely to respond with temper tantrums, crying episodes, or clinging behaviors. Reassure them that you will still be able to care for them, and keep them safe and well, despite the current situation. They are likely to manage better if you keep them informed with simple information.

Talk to your NICU team about the policies for sibling visitation. Brothers and sisters benefit from visiting the NICU. Rarely are they overwhelmed by the sights and sounds that bother adults. They tend to focus on the little human being whom they, too, have been expecting. Actually seeing the baby and the place that is the NICU, along with updates about your baby's progress, will help make the baby real and allow siblings to feel involved.

Alliyah gets involved by reading to **Eliana** in the NICU.

Involving Grandparents

You may have wonderful, supportive relationships with both sets of grandparents, who step up to the task and help you through the NICU experience with barely any coaching from you. Other NICU parents do not have such great relationships with their own parents and should think carefully about their own needs before inviting their parents to actively participate. If relationships are strained even before the baby comes along, the pressure of NICU care may add layers of stress. Some grandparents think they are being helpful by taking charge, but are actually doing things that are not helpful to the baby's parents. These grandparents may be surprised at first, but telling them what you really want them to do will pay off. Part of successful family relationships is knowing when to ask family members for help and support and when to ask them to give you space and let you make important decisions for yourself.

Friends

Friends can be a source of stress as well as support. If they fear saying the wrong thing, they may cope by avoiding you and the NICU experience at a time when their support would be helpful. Pregnant friends may feel guilty for being pregnant or having a healthy baby. Just when you need their support, they seem to pull away. This avoidance reflects your friends' feelings of inadequacy, rather than lack of caring. If you feel awkward or do not have the energy to do so, a steadfast friend, your partner, or your parents or partner's parents can tell your friends exactly what you need or how they can help. Friends usually have to be told only once, and then they'll make dinner, pick up your children at child care, run errands, or help in other directed ways.

> 66 In the beginning, you are in such a daze and everyone wants to come visit. I wish I had said no initially—to give us time to get used to our new normal. 99
>
> *Kate, mother of **Lucy***

Keeping Others Informed

There are many ways to keep family members and friends updated on your baby's progress, including all the ups and downs of a NICU course. Some strategies include assigning a person close to you to check in and distribute the messages or information that you choose to share via social media sites. Some hospitals have services that support development of a web page or an update page just for patients and families; these can be easy to build and are secure, and you invite only those you wish to view them. Ask the staff in your NICU about what is available and what has worked for other families. Be cautious about over sharing personal information online, such as your baby's full name, date and time of birth, parent names, city of birth, etc. It is unfortunate, but this information can be used by criminals to steal your child's identity.

> " Nurses were so kind and patient and encouraged us to become part of a care team and advocate for our babies. If my mom instinct was telling me something, they would bring my concerns to the doctors so they could be addressed. "
>
> *Parina, mother of* ***Isaac*** *and* ***Eliza***

Support Groups

Sources of support include extended family members, friends, nurses, social workers, the NICU staff, and other NICU parents. You may find that as your needs change over time, so do your support people.

At some point in your NICU stay, you may have questions that can only be answered by someone who has been through the experience. These questions can often be addressed in support groups that are offered at the hospital or in your community. Ask the NICU team if there is a parent-to-parent program or support group available in your area.

Understanding Your Baby

You may be concerned about your baby's ability to use all 5 senses. What are your baby's capabilities? How can you understand what your baby is telling you? Every baby is different, and your baby's gestational age at birth and health problems may influence the answers. The following descriptions apply to many babies in the NICU.

Vision

At the time of birth, babies born before 25 weeks of gestation often have eyelids that are fused closed. If your baby is born with closed eyelids, no special treatment is necessary. Your baby's eyes will open on their own within about 1 week of birth.

There is something very real and magical about looking into your baby's eyes. Parents in the NICU are often overheard saying, "Open your eyes, so I can see you and say hello." Looking into your baby's eyes can be a really special way to connect with your baby.

Position your baby face-to-face about 6 to 10 inches away. This is where your baby can see the best, and faces are a baby's favorite thing to look at. Initially, your baby may not be able to look at you and follow your face, but as your baby grows and remains awake for longer periods, this skill will improve.

A blanket over the incubator helps block bright light so your baby can rest.

Hearing

The ears begin to develop in the fourth week of gestation, and the sense of hearing continues to develop until the baby reaches term. As fetuses grow during pregnancy, they are exposed to a variety of sounds, such as their parent's heartbeat. Babies can recognize their parents' voices and may open their eyes and become alert or turn toward their parents when they speak. Some parents find it helpful to provide audio recordings with soothing sounds, such as soft music or their own voices reading or talking. Many NICU staff find that parents' voice recordings help the baby quiet and settle down to sleep.

Smell and Taste

The receptors in the nose and on the tongue used to detect smell and taste develop early in pregnancy. Even very preterm babies have a well-developed sense of smell and taste. Familiar smells and tastes may be comforting for your baby. When feeding, babies may prefer the taste of their parent's milk and recognize their parents' unique odor. Some NICUs give parents small cloth pads to wear and then place them in bed with their baby. This may comfort the baby and help the baby recognize the familiar smell in anticipation of breastfeeding.

Touch

The sense of touch also develops very early in gestation. Preterm babies can feel cloth against their skin and the warmth of their parents' skin against their own. Your baby's face, the area around the lips, and the hands are especially sensitive to your touch. Touching your baby is a wonderful way to connect and help care for your baby. You can help quiet your baby with a firm touch or by holding your baby's hand. Sometimes, babies are annoyed by stroking with your fingertips, perhaps because it feels like a tickle. As you touch your baby, watch the response and see what kind of touch helps your baby relax.

Your baby can feel pain, and pain control is an important part of NICU care. Nurses know to watch for signs of discomfort, such as facial expressions and increased heart rate, respiratory rate, blood pressure, and oxygen use. Ask your NICU team what strategies are being used to help keep your baby comfortable, as well as what you can do to help.

In addition to touching your baby, you can help create a sense of security by providing boundaries. Inside the uterus, your baby was surrounded and contained by the uterine wall. You can provide comfort in the same way by placing your warm hands against your baby's feet and on top of the head or by gently holding your baby's hands across the chest. The NICU staff can show you different ways to "contain" your baby, and you will learn what your baby likes best.

Babies also like a "nest," made of soft surfaces, as they lie in bed. Some units use special buntings or sleeping bags to provide *containment,* or they may place soft rolled blankets around your baby. Although these nesting materials are sometimes used in the NICU, by the time your baby is ready to go home, they are not necessary and should not be used. Unless your baby has medical needs for a special sleep position, your baby will sleep flat on the back on a firm mattress without any extra bedding or blankets before discharge, and this will continue at home.

Lukas and **Gabbie** calm with their dad's firm touch.

Babies appreciate boundaries. This father can calm his baby by gently holding the baby's arms and legs securely against his body.

Holland's mother provides secure boundaries by touching Holland's head and snuggling Holland's arms to her chest.

Alex feels secure in his "nest."

Your Baby's Personality

As babies in the NICU grow and continue to get stronger, their personalities begin to show. Before long, you will become aware of your baby's unique personality and methods of communicating likes and dislikes. To understand your baby's behavior, it is helpful to understand infant behavioral states and cues.

Deep sleep. The baby is very difficult to awaken from deep sleep.

Light sleep. The baby may move around, even fuss a little, in this state, but she is not fully awake.

Drowsy. The baby may open and close her eyes and move her arms and legs. By holding her upright and talking to her, you may be able to alert her. If left alone, she may go back to sleep.

Quiet alert. The baby "brightens" and focuses on your face or voice. As your preterm baby matures, her quiet alert periods will increase.

Active alert. The baby is alert but may become fussy and overwhelmed. If you decrease stimulation, she may recover and return to a quiet alert state.

Crying. She may calm down if held securely in quiet surroundings, given a pacifier or her fingers to suck on, or fed if she is hungry.

Behavioral States

Newborns experience 6 different levels of awareness called *behavioral states*. These states influence how a baby responds to the people and the environment. An ill or preterm baby will exhibit the same behavioral states as a healthy term baby, but these states may not be as easily recognized and the transition from state to state may not be as smooth.

Deep Sleep

In deep sleep, babies breathe regularly, their eyes are closed, and there are no noticeable eye movements. They do not move much but may startle or jerk. During deep sleep, your baby is difficult to arouse, does not respond to most stimulation, and is not interested in eating.

Light Sleep

In light sleep, also known as *rapid eye movement* or *REM sleep,* babies may breathe irregularly. Their eyes remain closed, but eye movements can be seen beneath the lids. Some activities, such as sucking movements, are common in light sleep. Your baby may fuss during this state and can be awakened enough to feed. This state is seen more clearly beginning at 36 weeks' gestation.

Drowsy

In the drowsy state, babies may open their eyes, or their eyelids may flutter. Babies may move their arms and legs, and their breathing may become rapid and shallow. If you hold your baby upright and speak, your baby may move from drowsiness into the quiet alert state but will go back to sleep if left alone.

Quiet Alert

In the quiet alert state, babies have a "bright" look and are able to focus their attention. This is the ideal state for parents to interact with their baby. Preterm babies can reach the quiet alert state but, often, only for a few seconds. As your baby matures, the periods of quiet alertness will increase.

Active Alert

Reacting to sound, touch, or movement, babies in the active alert state may startle and thrust their arms and legs. Their breathing can be irregular, they may be fussy, and they may not be able to focus their attention for very long. If you continue to speak or try to make eye contact at this time, your baby may start to cry. If you decrease the stimulation and offer rest and containment, your baby may relax and return to the quiet alert state.

Crying

Crying babies have exhausted their coping skills. In this state, babies need to rest or they need relief from pain, discomfort, or hunger.

Colson is in a quiet alert state and focuses on his mother's voice and face.

Behavioral Cues

When you learn to recognize your baby's state, you will begin to recognize the best times to interact and play.

Invitation Cues

These cues say, "I'm ready." Your baby will usually show invitation cues in the quiet alert state.

Baby Invitation Cues
▪ Bright look
▪ Relaxing hands, arms, legs
▪ Bringing hands to mouth
▪ Sucking on fingers, fist, or pacifier
▪ Making an "ooh" face by pursing lips
▪ Smiling or cooing
▪ Looking eye to eye, listening, watching your face

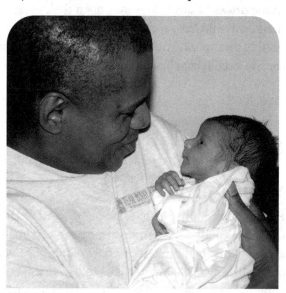

This baby is in a quiet alert state. He encourages his father to continue the interaction with invitation cues, such as his bright expression, good eye contact, and relaxed hand position.

Stress Cues

Not only will babies tell you when they are ready to interact, but they will tell you when they have had enough or are not in the mood. Babies show stress cues when they become tired or uncomfortable. Sometimes, your baby simply needs a short break, while other times your baby is telling you it's time to decrease stimulation, stop interacting for now, or go to sleep.

Baby Stress Cues

- Startling, jerking, or twitching
- Coughing, sneezing, yawning, or sighing
- Hiccupping, gagging, or grunting
- Squirming, turning away, arching
- Frantic or disorganized activity

This baby is signaling a need for a break by closing her eyes, turning her head away, and splaying her fingers.

This same baby displays increasing skill at self-comforting by flexing her arms to her midline and bracing her feet.

This baby's closed eyes, frowning face, stiff arms, and squirming body are clear stress signals. If swaddled and given total quiet, she may recover a quieter state.

Mixed Messages

Your baby may demonstrate a mixture of cues. For example, your baby may appear to be in the quiet alert state, ready to interact, yet at the same time be hiccupping. This mixture of cues can be frustrating and confusing. Do you act on the invitation to interact, or do you stop what you are doing and give your baby a break?

If your baby is sending out mixed messages, look for other cues to help you decide whether to interact. For example, if your baby has sent out several invitation cues but then spits up, your baby may have just finished eating and needed to burp. After burping (which caused the spit-up), your baby is again ready for interaction. If, on the other hand, your baby burps and begins to look tired and turns away from you, it's probably time for rest. With practice and experience, you'll learn what your baby is telling you in different situations.

Over time, your baby will use all 5 senses (touch, sound, smell, sight, and taste) to recognize you. At the same time, you will recognize what your baby likes and dislikes. Share with your NICU team the cues you see and what you learn about your baby. For instance, you may notice that your baby sleeps better on the right side or spits up less when held upright after feeding. These things are subtle but important parts of your baby's care.

Connecting With Your Baby

Babies and children learn through interacting with others. In the beginning, this interaction may be considered "playing" with your baby, and play is often seen as easy, natural, and requiring little thought. However, learning to play with your preterm or hospitalized baby may take some time. Initially, you may feel awkward, but as you become more familiar with your baby and see positive responses, you will look forward to your time together.

Eliana's dad is building confidence as he participates in her care.

> I finally started changing diapers and holding them. It felt good to be part of the team and contribute to their care.

*Parina, mother of **Isaac** and **Eliza***

One Thing at a Time

Follow your baby's lead. If your baby is showing invitation cues, start by allowing your baby to look at your face or hear your voice. *Try to introduce only one thing at a time.* Speaking into a

baby's face is instinctive for most of us, but it makes the baby look *and* listen. Speak to your baby first, and then watch for the reaction. Upon hearing your voice, your baby's eyes may brighten and your baby's head may turn to find you. At that point, your baby is ready to see your face. If your baby is very preterm or ill, seeing a face and hearing a voice or hearing your voice and being touched at the same time may be too much stimulation. You may quickly see your baby show some stress cues. Often, babies will gradually learn to handle more interaction and simultaneous stimulation as they grow, mature, and become more medically stable.

This baby connects with her mother by making eye contact and grasping her finger. Most preterm newborns can sustain this interaction only briefly, but these moments are enriching for the baby and rewarding for her parents.

Courtesy of Gigi O'Dea.

> Regardless of how much time you're able to spend in the NICU, make it count. Put your phone away, hold your baby skin to skin, and get to know your baby. This helps you build a strong bond, it helps you learn about your baby's personality and moods and patterns, and it prepares you for life outside the NICU.
>
> *Kate and Matt, parents of **Lucy***

Nonnutritive Sucking

Another important learning activity for babies is nonnutritive sucking. This type of sucking does not provide nutrition; rather, babies suck on their own finger or thumb, on a pacifier, on your clean finger, or at a breast after pumping. Nonnutritive sucking helps babies comfort themself and "organize" their behavioral states, gain weight, improve their feeding skills, and decrease their oxygen needs.

Using a pacifier helps **Eliana** stay calm, gain weight, improve feeding skills, and decrease oxygen needs.

Positioning

Positioning may be used to help your baby stay calm, focused, and "organized" in the different behavioral states. Term newborns prefer to curl up in a flexed position, but preterm newborns may not be able to flex their limbs and keep them flexed without assistance. Flexing your baby forward and bringing your baby's arms and legs to the center of the body can help your baby discover comfort behaviors, such as finger or hand sucking. Body containment, by swaddling and nesting, helps your baby feel safe and secure and promotes normal growth and development. Your NICU team will teach you how to hold and position your baby properly.

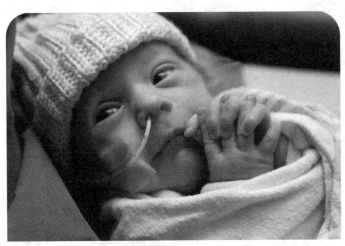

This baby is swaddled just enough to contain his arms and legs. His hands are outside the blanket and centered so that he can bring them together and suck his hands or fingers. *Courtesy of Gigi O'Dea.*

Skin-to-Skin Care (Kangaroo Care)

Ask your baby's NICU team when you can hold your baby skin-to-skin, which is called *kangaroo care* in some NICUs. Kangaroo care was developed in South America to keep preterm newborns warm. Mothers were instructed to hold their diapered preterm newborns skin-to-skin beneath their clothing for warmth and breastfeeding. While many NICUs now call the practice *skin-to-skin care,* the term *kangaroo care* has been affectionately maintained in some units.

Both parents can participate in skin-to-skin care. Most nurseries have comfortable chairs and privacy screens that can be placed around your chair or the baby's care area. Simply wear clothing that opens down the front. You will snuggle your baby upright on your chest or lay your baby's head against your chest.

The benefits of skin-to-skin care for the newborn include warmth, stability of heartbeat and breathing, increased time spent in the deep sleep and quiet alert states, decreased crying, increased weight gain, and improved breastfeeding. These benefits occur even when skin-to-skin care occurs for only a few minutes each day. At a time when so many people are caring for your baby, skin-to-skin care provides special moments of closeness and comfort that only you can experience with your baby.

Skin-to-Skin (Kangaroo) Care

Skin-to-skin care is a fundamental expression of parenting. It is important and beneficial for both parents and their baby, too.

A short time after **Abel's** birth, he and his dad were able to snuggle with kangaroo care.

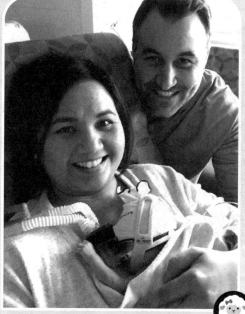

Eliana, who has graduated to CPAP in this photo, continues to benefit from skin-to-skin care.

Alex's parents took turns doing skin-to-skin care. They both felt this experience helped them bond with their infant son.

Meridith, 2 days old, gets to know her dad.

Growing With Your Baby

During the NICU stay, you'll notice how your baby is growing—physically as well as developmentally. During that time, parents will grow as well. Celebrate accomplishments and "firsts": the first time you hold, bathe, or feed your baby. You may wish to capture these moments in a special collection of photos and memories that mark progress during your baby's NICU stay. Enjoy the special time you have with your baby. Although this is probably not the way you had imagined becoming acquainted, it can be a memorable and special experience.

Logan

Born at 34 weeks

Our visit to the university neonatal intensive care unit (NICU) was totally unexpected so it did not come with anticipation, nervousness, or anxiety. We were blessed to have many wonderful doctors and nurses to help us through everything with as little stress as possible. I hope that sharing my memories can help with your journey. This is my story.

It was a normal work day at the office when I felt something odd in my tummy. It was the end of August and I was not due until the second week in October so I knew something was wrong. In hindsight I now know that this was our baby, nicknamed Nester, letting me know labor had begun. This process would have been covered in our Lamaze training if we had made it that far in the program, but Nester had other ideas. I immediately left the office and started planning my next steps during the 45-minute, pain-stricken ride home. I finally got a call back from my husband, Tom, who would meet me at home where we would call triage and then make our way to the hospital.

Upon arrival at triage, I was told I was dilated (at 1 cm), continued to have contractions, and was admitted to the hospital where we waited, and waited, and waited. Nester decided that he was very comfortable exactly where he was! Twenty-four hours later my labor had not progressed so the doctors decided to administer an intravenous drug that would help stop contractions and sent me home. I rested at home the next day, but no matter how much medicine I took I could not get rid of a terrible headache. We called our fabulous doctor friend who told us to immediately call triage.

Back in the hospital I was diagnosed with preeclampsia, which is a pregnancy complication that can include high blood pressure, swelling of hands and feet, accumulation of fluids, and protein spilled in urine. My agonizing headache was alerting my body to my dangerously high blood pressure. My original birthing plan included listening to soothing music, using my Lamaze positions to ease my baby through the birth canal, and using no pain medication—a beautiful affair that would gently bring Nester into our world. Thus far the birth was not going accordingly to my plan. The new plan consisted of me laying stationary in a hospital bed, getting 2 very painful shots 24 hours apart to help develop Nester's lungs, getting a drip of magnesium sulfate, and having my blood pressure checked every hour. Needless to say, I was exhausted well before it was time to push. Did I mention that neither of the attempts for an epidural reacted properly with my body? If I had known what I had to conquer prior to delivering Nester, I would have been terrified, but in the moment, there was nothing I would not do to keep Nester safe. There is no fear, just action. There was one point during pushing that I thought, "I cannot do this. How can I possibly

Logan's parents, Tom and Christina, spent 7 days with Logan in the NICU.

keep pushing?" and then my body just kept pushing. Once the oxytocin kicked in, Nester was born so quickly. It was a beautiful miracle and the most amazing thing I had ever accomplished.

Nester, now officially named Logan, was a precious baby boy delivered at 34 weeks, weighing 5 pounds 7 ounces and 18.3 inches long. He was the most perfect baby I had ever seen. I was allowed to hold Logan for only a few minutes before he was rushed to the NICU. It was such a blur and my husband and I had no idea what to do. The doctors were still stitching me up when I firmly told him to follow our baby wherever he went, as I would be okay. At that time, I had no idea there was an intensive care unit for babies because I never thought about mothers having complicated births. In my mind all mothers gave birth, sent their children to the nursery, and then everyone went home safely 2 days later.

I was required to continue with the magnesium sulfate drip and get my hourly blood pressure taken for 24 hours after giving birth. I couldn't leave my hospital bed but I was aching to visit my baby. My fabulous nurse rolled my entire hospital bed up to the NICU and I held Logan's hand for the first time! My husband was there when Logan was hooked up to a breathing machine and feeding tube and put in an incubator but it was quite shocking and overwhelming to me. I wanted to wrap my arms around Logan and embrace his tiny body but I couldn't with all of his tubes and attachments.

After visiting the NICU for the first time, I realized that Logan was one of the largest patients admitted at the time. Logan was only 6 weeks early, which is nothing compared to some of the very premature babies in the NICU. Still, so many different thoughts were running through my head: What if I hurt him? Would he be okay? Why did he need all of this equipment? Was I not a good mother housing him for only 34 weeks? What did I do wrong? But mostly I was exhausted and I had lost a lot of blood. Our doctor friend came to visit while she was doing rounds and suggested I get back to bed and rest. I wanted to stay with Logan so badly but needed to leave to take care of myself.

While I was recovering, I missed his first feeding, first diaper change, first bath, etc. It was really difficult to know that my premature baby was only 2 floors away but I could not get to him. Tom was struggling with supporting both of us, trying to be in 2 places at once. He did not want to miss one moment of being with Logan nor did he want to leave me alone with a tough recovery. He was in an impossible situation but did a great job of moving between us frequently. Even though I was often away from Logan, the nurses tried to keep me as involved as possible. After Logan's first bath I received a note from a nurse apologizing for bathing him without me. On a different occasion I received a card "from Logan" saying how much he missed me. The nurses were so cognizant that normally a family would be having these firsts together and did everything they could to be sensitive to the situation. I was so impressed with the positive attitudes and enthusiastic energy of all the doctors, nurses, and support staff encountered during a difficult time for our family.

After a 7-day stay in the NICU, Tom and I were allowed to take Logan home! I was so looking forward to going home and getting our lives started but also terrified that we would be on our own. The nurses sent us on our way with everything not nailed down in the room, which made me feel a little better about making it on our own. While finally leaving the hospital, Tom brought the car around and I delicately placed the baby carrier into the car attachment. I climbed in the car beside Logan and was so proud of all we had already gone through as a family.

Five-year old Logan is learning to read.

As we pulled away, "All My Love" by Led Zeppelin started playing and I was overcome with a sense of calm, knowing we would all be okay.

It has been almost 6 crazy, messy, fabulous years since Logan came into our lives. He has grown into a very tall, very active 5-year-old who loves drawing, nature, and animals. He is currently deciding if he will be a geologist or botanist when he grows up. Logan is smart, funny, and creative. He is one of my favorite people and I could not imagine life without him.

Tom and Christina, parents of Logan

Maxwell

Born at 34 weeks
· · · · · · · · · · · · · ·

Our 22-day stay in the NICU was a nerve-racking, challenging time. We went from being at home preparing for baby, to emergency C-section and not knowing if our baby would survive, to living in the hospital with a 5½-pound newborn who was struggling to breathe, suck, and swallow and maintain his body temperature. Looking back now, it was truly amazing to see him develop and grow before our eyes and get stronger each day. We were growing as parents too. We were kind of thrown into the deep end of the pool, paddling to survive.

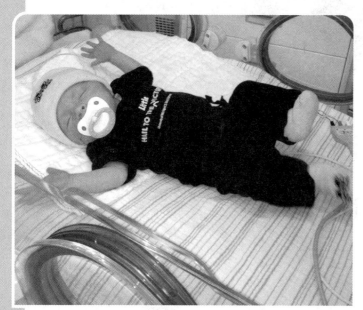

Maxwell in his going-home outfit.

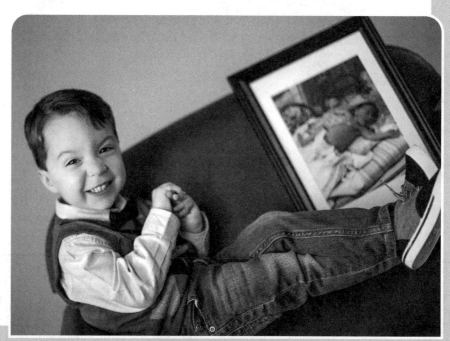

Maxwell, at age 3 years, sitting next to his NICU photo.

The NICU is an amazing place where amazing medicine happens. It can also be an extremely lonely place. Without the empathy and compassion from the doctors and nurses, I'm not sure how anyone could survive those first few weeks.

Maxwell is a healthy 3-year-old today. He still has underdeveloped lungs and gets infections like croup quite often. He also had some delays. He didn't walk until 18 months and he didn't get all of his baby teeth until age 3.

We are so proud of our little man and look forward to all of the great things he will accomplish in his life.

Amanda and Gabriel, parents of Maxwell

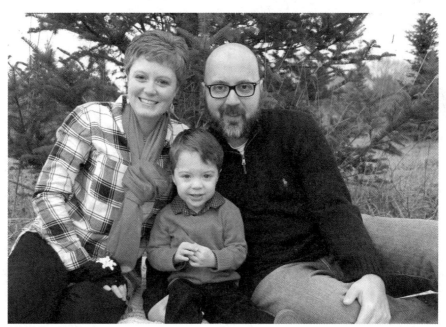

Maxwell and his parents.

CHAPTER 7

Feeding Your Baby

> Feeding Eliana by bottle was challenging at first because she had to learn to breathe while she was sucking. We constantly watched the monitor to make sure her numbers weren't dropping until our nurse told us to stop looking at the monitor and just look at our baby for cues, because at home we wouldn't have a monitor to look at. That helped us relax a bit and just enjoy feeding our baby!
>
> *Sophany and Mike, parents of **Eliana***

Feeding your baby is an important parenting task and a satisfying activity you will want to share with your baby; however, right after birth, your baby may not be able to feed directly from the breast or bottle. Many babies in the neonatal intensive care unit (NICU) will receive nourishment in different ways for some period of time.

Your Baby's First Nutrition

· · · · · · · · · · · · · · · · ·

You may be amazed at how hard your tiny newborn can suck on your finger or a pacifier shortly after birth, but it doesn't mean your baby is ready to begin breastfeeding or bottle-feeding. Criteria for oral feeding vary among units, but, commonly, babies in the NICU will start oral feeding attempts when they are clinically stable, breathing without difficulty, and displaying oral feeding cues. Frequently, this occurs when preterm babies are close to 32 to 34 weeks' gestation but the timing may vary for any individual baby. Once babies start oral feeding attempts, it may be a while before they have the skills to suck, swallow, and breathe in a coordinated way. Feeding a sick or preterm baby in the NICU can be a slow and deliberate process, with potential complications. Until breastfeeding or bottle-feeding is safe, your baby will be nourished in other ways.

Intravenous Nutrition

Your baby may not be fed by mouth immediately after birth. Instead, nutrition may be provided through an *intravenous line* (*IV*) placed in one of your baby's veins. If your baby is very preterm or will not be able to begin feedings for several days, *total parenteral nutrition* (*TPN*) may be used. *Parenteral* refers to nutrition that enters the body through a blood vessel, while *enteral* refers to nutrition that enters the body through the stomach and intestines. Using TPN, your baby can receive all the essential nutrients (sugar, protein, fat, vitamins, and minerals) through an IV.

Tube Feeding

Babies can suck long before they are able to coordinate the process of sucking, swallowing, and breathing. They get their breast milk (sometimes called *human milk*) or formula through a *feeding tube* inserted through the nose or mouth and advanced into the stomach. Tube feeding is occasionally called *gavage* feeding. The most common methods of tube feeding use a soft tube passed through the mouth into the baby's stomach (an *orogastric* tube) or a tube passed through the nose into the stomach (a *nasogastric* tube). Occasionally, the tube will be advanced further into the baby's intestine (*orojejunal* or *nasojejunal* tube). Giving your baby a pacifier to suck on during tube feeding may encourage the development and coordination of sucking skills, improve weight gain, and shorten the time to full oral feedings.

To start, your baby may receive very small amounts of breast milk or formula. These small feedings are intended to get the baby's stomach and intestines ready to absorb nutrients. Your baby may receive milk on a regular schedule, such as every 2 or 3 hours (*intermittent tube feeding*) or may receive milk from a pump that provides a steady slow flow through the tube (*continuous* tube feeding). Intermittent tube feeding given rapidly may be called *bolus* feeding. Babies who are tube fed are carefully watched to make sure they are tolerating the feedings. The baby is watched for bloating (*distention*) of the abdomen and for vomiting.

As your baby becomes ready, the amount of milk provided will gradually increase. The NICU dietitian may also recommend adding calories, minerals, and vitamins to the milk with a liquid or powder fortifier. As the amount of milk is increased, the amount of IV fluid or TPN is slowly decreased. When your baby is taking enough milk to support healthy growth, sometimes called *full feeds*, the IV may be removed, unless it is still needed for medications.

When measuring fluids and weights, the NICU team often uses the more accurate metric system. You will hear fluid described in milliliters (mL) and weight described in grams (g) or kilograms (kg). For your reference, 1 ounce (oz) is 28 mL (some NICUs count 1 oz as equal to 30 mL to make calculations easier) and 1 kg is 2.2 pounds (lb). Depending on your baby's age and medical condition, full feeds require your baby to take about 120 to 150 mL of milk per kilogram of body weight each day (just about 2 to 2½ oz per pound per day). The Appendix contains a chart to help you convert grams to pounds and ounces.

Ensuring Adequate Nutrition

Gaining and Growing

After birth, weight gain and growth are closely watched to ensure good nutrition, which affects brain growth and the ability to learn physical, social, and emotional skills (*developmental outcome*). Your NICU team will plot your baby's growth—weight, length, and head circumference changes—on growth charts.

Weight Gain, Length, and Head Circumference

Babies in the NICU are weighed daily or every few days, depending on their health status. After birth, babies are expected to lose some weight. During the first week after birth, term babies may lose up to 7% to 10% of their birth weight; preterm babies may lose up to 12% to 15%. For example, if your baby is preterm, weighs 1,200 g at birth, and loses 15% of birth weight, your baby's weight would fall to 1,020 g (15% of 1,200 g is 180 g).

Term babies usually lose weight only for the first few days after birth. Preterm newborns may lose weight for longer than a few days before starting to gain it back. Once your baby starts gaining weight, it may take some time to establish a regular pattern. Even when your baby does begin to gain weight regularly, there will be occasional days of no gain or even a slight loss. Because of the day-to-day variation, most NICU teams assess a growing baby's average weight gain over a week to follow the trend.

Growth Goals

When your baby is in stable condition and can use energy for growth, the average daily expected weight gain is about 15 to 20 g for each kilogram of body weight. When your baby approaches discharge, the goal for weight gain is about 15 to 30 g per day or about ½ to 1 oz per day.

Your baby's body length and head size (*circumference*) are also important and will be measured periodically. Increase in a healthy baby's head circumference usually means brain growth. Overall, the goal is to increase length and head circumference by about 1 cm (a little less than ½ inch) per week.

"" After 53 days in the NICU, progress continues slowly but surely, but, unfortunately, with no end in sight. I can't complain much because both girls are doing so well, but I must admit that the long haul is starting to take its toll emotionally. I've always liked the quote, 'If it doesn't kill you, it makes you stronger.' Well, if that's true, I should be one tough cookie by the end of this! ""

*Billie, mother of **Holland** and **Eden***

Benefits of Breast Milk

For most babies in the NICU, breast milk is the best choice because it provides protection from infections, allergies, and other diseases. Providing breast milk for your sick or preterm baby is perhaps the most important thing you can do for your baby's health. If expressed milk from the birthing parent is not available, your baby may be offered donor breast milk (see Can I Use Donated Breast Milk for My Baby? later in this chapter), which is a very good option. If necessary, babies in the NICU can be fed formula made from cow's milk or soybeans, but for most NICU babies, formula cannot provide the benefits they receive from breast milk.

Benefits of Breast Milk

- Breast milk after premature delivery differs from that produced after a full-term pregnancy and has more of the nutrients, such as protein, that a preterm baby needs. However, the composition of breast milk changes over time and becomes similar to term milk within a few weeks. It is often necessary to add nutritional components to breast milk (*fortify breast milk*) to ensure complete nutrition for preterm infants.

- Nutrients in breast milk are absorbed more easily than the nutrients in formula made from cow's milk or soybeans.

- Feeding preterm newborns breast milk decreases the risk of a serious intestinal illness (*necrotizing enterocolitis*) and eye disease (*retinopathy of prematurity*).

- Developmental outcomes in preterm newborns are improved by feeding breast milk.

- Breast milk contains substances that protect a baby from infection. Breastfeeding decreases the risk of ear infections, diarrhea, and serious colds.

- Breastfeeding reduces the risk of sudden infant death syndrome (SIDS), allergies and asthma, celiac disease, inflammatory bowel disease, obesity, type 1 diabetes mellitus (often called juvenile-onset diabetes), and childhood leukemia.

When Not to Use Breast Milk or Breastfeed

Most babies benefit from the parent's milk; however, in some situations, it may not be safe for your baby to breastfeed or receive breast milk. Babies with a rare metabolic disease called *galactosemia* should not receive breast milk. In the United States, it is recommended that parents with HIV not breastfeed or give their baby their breast milk since the virus may be transferred to the infant through the milk. Direct breastfeeding should not occur if the parent has untreated active tuberculosis or has active herpes lesions on their breasts; however, expressed milk can be used because there is no concern about these infectious organisms passing through the milk. There are some medications and supplements that make breast milk unsafe, so you should let your NICU team know about all drugs and dietary supplements the breastfeeding parent is consuming. In addition, the use of expressed breast milk and breastfeeding may need to be stopped or limited for parents who are drinking alcohol or using other potentially harmful substances such as amphetamines, ecstasy, cocaine, or heroin. More information is provided about these substances later in this chapter.

Can I Use Donated Breast Milk for My Baby?

The evidence is clear that breast milk is beneficial for the health and development of babies, and many NICUs strive to give preterm and ill babies only breast milk. Doing so sometimes requires the use of donated breast milk from a milk bank. The American Academy of Pediatrics recommends using the parent's milk whenever possible, but if the parent's milk is not available, pasteurized donor milk is the next best choice. The United States and Canada have a growing number of milk banks supervised by the Human Milk Banking Association of North America (HMBANA). Milk banks screen donors to make sure they are healthy and do not have diseases that could be transmitted in their milk. The individuals who donate to HMBANA milk banks are volunteers who do not get paid for their generous gift. The milk is gently heated and pasteurized to destroy bacteria, while preserving most of the milk's important qualities. The milk is tested for bacterial growth and when it passes its quality testing, it is frozen and shipped to hospitals and individuals who need it. If donor milk is used for your infant, it should come from a certified milk bank to ensure your baby's health and safety and not from friends, neighbors, or the internet.

The process of obtaining donor milk varies among hospitals. In many hospitals, a medical order and parental consent are needed to use donor breast milk. At this time, it costs about $4.50 per ounce—more expensive than most formula, but inexpensive compared to its potential benefits. Some hospitals pay the extra cost for donor milk from a regulated milk bank, but many do not. Your insurance or Medicaid may not cover the cost either. Talk with your NICU team about using donated milk if you cannot provide all the milk your baby needs. It is well worth the effort to give your preterm baby breast milk.

If a Parent Has Had Breast Surgery

Breast implants usually do not interfere with breastfeeding unless breast damage occurred from the surgery. Breast reduction always affects milk production, but parents may be able to produce some milk depending on the type of surgery performed. Talk with your baby's lactation specialist about the type of breast surgery and what you can expect.

Providing Breast Milk for Your Baby

Providing breast milk for your baby is one of the most important things you can do for your baby's health. Every family has a lot to think about after labor and birth. Amid all the activity, be sure to tell your caregivers that you are planning to breastfeed your baby.

How the Breasts Make Milk

To appreciate the importance of pumping your breasts often and completely, it helps to understand how breasts work.

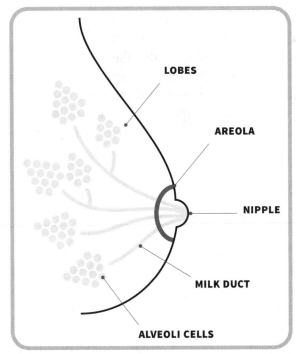

LOBES

AREOLA

NIPPLE

MILK DUCT

ALVEOLI CELLS

Milk production occurs within the milk glands (called alveoli) which are grape-like clusters of cells within the breast. In response to nursing or pumping, the milk is squeezed into the milk ducts, which carry the milk through the breast to the nipple.

Source: U.S. Department of Agriculture.

Shortly after the baby's birth, breasts start producing a thick clear or yellow-gold liquid called *colostrum*. Within 2 or 3 days after delivery, the colostrum begins to change to a thinner, whiter milk. On about day 3 or 4, hormones cause the breasts to become swollen, hard, and painful. When this happens, people may say that the "milk is coming in." This happens whether the baby is born early or at full term and whether the parent breastfeeds or not.

Milk can be expressed in 3 ways: by nursing the baby, by expressing milk manually (the parent uses their hands to squeeze milk from the breast), or by suctioning milk out with a breast pump.

Regardless of the manner in which milk is expressed, the brain releases 2 hormones. *Prolactin* causes the milk glands in the breasts to start secreting milk, and *oxytocin* causes contractions of tiny muscles that surround the milk glands (called alveoli, a different kind of alveoli than found in the lungs). These contractions squeeze the milk through the milk ducts to the nipples. This is called the *milk-ejection reflex* or the *letdown reflex*. An early sign that the letdown reflex is occurring may be menstrual-like cramps. These cramps are noticeable only in the first week or two after birth, and may not be noticeable at all if this is your first baby. After a week or so, the parent may notice the letdown reflex as a feeling of thirst a few minutes after beginning to pump, a tingling sensation or "pins and needles" in the breasts, or milk dripping from the nipples. After pumping, a distinct softening of the breasts is often noticed.

What to Expect in the First Few Days

Soon after a newborn is admitted to the NICU, the staff will provide a breast pump to the lactating parent. If the parent's medical condition allows, pumping within the first 6 hours after giving birth is ideal. The staff will explain how to hold the milk-collecting cups to the breasts and turn on the pump. At first, using the breast pump may feel awkward and embarrassing— and possibly discouraging when only a drop or two of milk appears on the nipple, but every drop is precious. This first milk is sometimes called "liquid gold." Save every drop in a small container. The volume of your baby's first feeding is very small, perhaps only 1 to 2 mL (about ¼ teaspoon).

Your first breast milk (colostrum) may be used for your baby's oral care and is sometimes called immunotherapy. This is the process of applying drops of colostrum into your baby's mouth by using a syringe (with no needle) or a cotton swab. This is not meant to provide nutrition and the baby does not need to swallow. Colostrum contains many immune agents that may be absorbed through the infant's gums, which can help decrease the risk of respiratory and gastrointestinal infections. This method of oral care also provides positive oral stimulation that may reduce the effects of negative oral experiences that can lead to oral aversion and feeding problems.

Trying to learn about pumping and storing milk in the first few hours after giving birth may feel overwhelming. This may not be the best time to take in new information. Don't be afraid to ask questions and repeat them until you understand the answers. Watch educational videos, if they are available, and ask for written materials to read on your own schedule. Arrange to have your partner, a family member, or a friend in the room when the NICU staff is explaining everything; chances are that between the 2 of you, you'll remember the important points.

> ❝ Stick with the pumping for as long as you possibly can. Work with the lactation consultants and your nurses and let them know you want to breastfeed—they are there to help you succeed. ❞
>
> *Kate, mother of **Lucy***

Pumping Breast Milk

This is a list of basic information. Your nurses and lactation specialist will provide you with more information.

- Pump both breasts 8 to 10 times a day for about 15 minutes at a time, even if only a drop or two comes out. The milk supply will often increase by the third to fifth day. To help open the ducts and increase milk flow, apply a warm, moist compress and gently massage the breast before and during pumping.

- Do not let the breasts feel full between pumping, as this can decrease milk supply. If you decide that sleep is more important than pumping, don't let more than 6 hours go by without pumping. Do not skip pumping at night very often.

- Do not use a small hand-operated or battery-powered pump. Only a hospital-quality, fully automatic electric pump is adequate for the job. Pump both breasts at the same time. This not only saves time but also increases prolactin levels. The hospital will have breast pumps for use while in the NICU. Ask about renting a hospital-grade pump for use at home. Your insurance or Medicaid may help with rental costs.

- Ask your NICU staff for advice about storing milk at home and how to bring milk to the NICU. You may pack it in a small cooler, or, for long-distance travel, you may be asked to pack it in dry ice in a sturdy, insulated container.

- Breast milk is not sterile, but it must stay clean. Clean the breast pump parts well, wash hands before pumping, and follow your NICU's instructions. If you are unsure about any cleaning or pumping procedures, ask for help.

- The NICU staff may provide printed labels or a bar code to use on the containers. They will check the label or scan the bar code before giving the milk to your baby to reduce the chance of giving your baby another parent's breast milk.

- Your NICU staff will teach you how to thaw and warm breast milk in the NICU and after your baby comes home.

- Continue to pump when the baby begins to breastfeed in the NICU. Ask the NICU team when to pump if you know which feeding times your baby will try breastfeeding.

Help Your Baby Get Ready for the Breast or Bottle

You can help your baby develop the oral feeding skills necessary for breastfeeding and bottle-feeding by using the following techniques:

Nonnutritive Sucking

Sucking that does not supply nutrition is called *nonnutritive sucking*. This is good sucking practice and helps with weight gain and digestion. Nonnutritive sucking also helps the baby develop self-calming skills.

Watch for signs that your baby would like to suck. Babies may show feeding cues, such as bringing their hand to their mouth, turning their head and opening their mouth, or making sucking motions. Nonnutritive sucking can occur if your preterm baby nuzzles at the parent's breast during skin-to-skin care (see Chapter 6). You can also slip your clean finger into your baby's mouth and gently stroke the roof of the mouth with the pad of your finger, or give your baby a pacifier to suck when awake and alert.

Abel is given the opportunity to use his pacifier to practice sucking and develop self-calming skills.

"**Reece** and **Allison** are 15 days old. They are receiving no respiratory assistance, their PICC lines have been removed, and they have overcome jaundice. They are still relying on their feeding tubes."

Gudrun, mother of Allison and Reece

Patience and Practice

Depending on your baby's gestational age and health, tube feeding may continue for several days, weeks, or even months. If you move too quickly to breastfeeding or bottle-feeding, your baby will use too much energy trying to eat and may get tired, have more breathing problems, lose weight, and have difficulty staying warm. The transition from tube feeding to breastfeeding or bottle-feeding can be frustrating for parents.

Your NICU team will assess your baby's health and feeding skills and work with you to decide when to try breastfeeding or bottle-feeding. Some NICUs have protocols for step-by-step increases in oral feeding attempts. Be patient. Some feedings will go well; others will be more difficult. Work with the NICU staff to find those times of day when your baby is most awake, alert, and showing signs of readiness to practice feeding by mouth.

Learning to breastfeed or bottle-feed takes time—it doesn't happen overnight. A growing preterm baby may feed well once but may not do so again for another day or longer. Many preterm babies can breastfeed well by the time they reach their full-term due date, but many will go home with a combination of breastfeeding and bottle-feeding.

> Once Sienna no longer needed assistance breathing, it seemed like she was ready to come home! She was bright-eyed and seemed to be looking at me, wondering why she had to stay. This was a difficult phase of the NICU. It was a waiting game, as she learned how to suck, swallow, and breathe at the same time. I got frustrated with the baby steps. Looking back, it was the absolute best thing in the world for her to have stayed there as long as she did.
>
> *Kaitlynn, mother of **Sienna***

Learning to Breastfeed

Learning to breastfeed is a skill for the breastfeeding parent and baby. Getting comfortable enough to nurse in the NICU adds a little more stress. Be patient and give yourself a lot of time to learn. Many babies in their early days seem to sleep through the experience. Your patience will pay off. Gradually, your baby will show more interest in nursing, and you will gain confidence with your skills.

The best way to learn to breastfeed your baby is to ask the nurse or lactation specialist to help you. They can answer your questions and help with another set of hands and arms until you can manage alone.

Here is a list of basic tips that may be helpful as you and your baby learn what works best for you.

▸ Sit in a comfortable chair and rest your feet on a small footstool.

▸ A pillow on your lap may help bring the baby level to your breast. Do not hunch over to nurse a baby in your lap.

▸ Two common positions for breastfeeding work especially well for preterm babies.

— **The cross-cradle hold:** Lay your baby sideways facing you, with the baby's mouth right beside your nipple. Encircle your baby's body with the arm opposite the breast that your baby is about to nurse from, and grasp the back of the baby's lower head, neck, and shoulder blades in your hand. With the same-side hand (for example, left hand on left breast), cup your breast by placing your 4 fingers underneath and your thumb on top of your breast.

— **The football or clutch hold:** Place your baby on a pillow with the baby's legs pointing toward the back of the chair or bed. The same hand as the side of the breast you plan to offer will support the baby's head, neck, and shoulder. The baby is brought up to the breast in a gentle motion toward the nipple. The opposite hand is used to lift and guide the breast for the baby.

The football or clutch hold works well for many preterm babies. Hold the baby at your side, with the baby's mouth in front of your breast and the baby's feet pointing toward your back. Your opposite hand supports the breast and guides the nipple into the baby's mouth.

Courtesy of Gigi O'Dea.

Shana uses a cross-cradle hold as **Abel** practices breastfeeding.

▶ Find a comfortable hand position for holding the breast as you offer the nipple to the baby and support your breast as your baby nurses. Your breast is most likely so heavy that it will pull out of the baby's mouth if you don't support it.

— With your fingers cupping your breast, press the dark area around the nipple (the *areola*) to fit your baby's mouth. Although the mouth forms a circle when open wide, as soon as it clamps onto your areola and nipple, the lips and gums form a flattened oval. If you gently compress your breast into that same oval shape, your baby is likely to be able to suck longer. Keep your thumb and fingers a little behind the areola so they are not in the way of your baby's mouth. Think about how you squeeze a very thick sandwich just before you take a bite or how you turn an oval peg to fit it into an oval hole. Be sure that your thumb is parallel to your baby's upper lip and your index finger is parallel to your baby's lower lip.

— Some parents find a U-shaped hold works better than a C-shaped hold to ensure the weight of the breast does not interfere with the baby's ability to suckle and for the hand to provide additional jaw support. The U-hold is achieved by placing the thumb on one side of the breast behind the areola, with other fingers placed on the opposite side. In other words, slide your fingers toward the center of your body and your thumb toward the outside of your breast.

— Stroke the center of your baby's lower lip with the tip of your nipple. Brush your nipple lightly over the lower lip, as if giving a signal. If you are able, express a few drops of milk to offer a familiar taste and smell. This can encourage a baby to open their mouth and search for the nipple. When your baby is older and more experienced, this technique of touching your baby's lip with your nipple will be a powerful cue—your baby may open their mouth wide. If your baby's mouth does not open, the lactation specialist or nurse can gently apply slight pressure to the chin to help your baby open wide or help to shape your nipple and aim it toward the roof of your baby's mouth.

▶ Then, with a forward movement of the arm encircling your baby, you'll guide the baby onto your breast. As you do so, aim your nipple up toward the roof of your baby's mouth. This helps ensure you get your nipple above your baby's tongue. Pull your baby in so close that the tip of the baby's nose touches your breast. Continue to gently compress and support the weight of your breast throughout the *entire* feeding.

Signs That Your Baby Is Properly Latching on to the Breast

- Your baby has a wide-open mouth with lips spread out around your breast.
- Your baby's mouth covers your entire nipple and some of the areola.
- You feel a firm tug on your breast every time your baby sucks.
- Your baby can suckle for more than 3 or 4 sucks in a row.
- Your baby can hang onto your nipple during pauses between bursts of sucks.

Is Your Baby Getting Milk?

Once your baby is latched on well, you may notice small, quick bursts of sucking until your milk begins to flow. Then the sucking pattern will change to slower, deeper, more rhythmic sucks. If the NICU is quiet, you may be able to hear your baby swallow. This is a sure sign that milk is flowing. If you cannot hear swallowing, look at your baby's neck for swallowing movement or ask the NICU staff to observe you breastfeeding and confirm that your baby is swallowing.

When you first begin to breastfeed, your *milk-ejection (letdown) reflex* may not occur until after your baby has tired of sucking and fallen asleep. But, just as your body became conditioned to respond to the breast pump, you will learn to respond to your baby's suck.

After a few minutes of sustained, rhythmic sucks, your baby may revert to bursts of little sucks with long pauses in between. The swallowing sounds will be further and further apart. It's time to take your baby off your breast (breastfeeding parents may need to break the suction with a full-term baby by putting their finger in the baby's mouth to interrupt sucking), burp your baby, and switch to the other breast. On the second side, watch again for the sucking pattern to slow down and for swallowing to become less frequent.

During early feedings, your preterm baby may not be able to tolerate this "burp and switch" technique. Taking your baby off the breast and switching back and forth may cause your baby to tire. Ask the NICU staff for advice about nursing on only one breast at a feeding.

Some NICUs weigh the baby (fully clothed) before and after a feeding to estimate how much milk the baby got during the feeding. Each gram of weight gain is equal to approximately 1 mL of milk. For example, if your baby gained 15 g after a feeding, your baby took about 15 mL (½ oz). If your NICU uses this method to estimate intake, ask when the process begins.

This baby seems alert and begins this feeding at the breast. When he tires, the remainder of the feeding will be given through his feeding tube.

Courtesy of Gigi O'Dea.

At first, your baby may be able to breastfeed only once or twice a day. Growing preterm babies become tired and may lose weight if you push them to nurse more than they are able. Continue to pump immediately after each nursing session to maintain your milk supply. Although it's tempting to say, "I breastfed the baby, so I don't need to pump," if you don't keep pumping after every breastfeeding, you risk losing your milk supply.

Supportive Care for Breastfeeding Parents

Breastfeeding is a big commitment and requires a considerable amount of supportive care. Your NICU team, including the lactation specialist, may offer more information about ways to make sure a breastfeeding parent stays healthy. The following information will get you started and may prompt you to think of additional questions.

Diet

A healthy pregnancy diet should continue after the baby is born. Breastfeeding parents need to make good choices, listen to their body, and eat when they're hungry. It is important to include a variety of proteins, fats, and carbohydrates. Ask your health care professional if continuing to take a prenatal vitamin or a nutritional supplement is recommended. If you have questions about a healthy diet, ask your health care professional or your baby's dietitian for suggestions.

Fluids

Breastfeeding parents should drink about 8 glasses of fluid—which should be mostly water— every 24 hours. This is not difficult for most breastfeeding people because each time they pump or nurse they will feel thirsty. They should drink whenever they are thirsty and keep the color of their urine a clear yellow, not cloudy or a dark yellow.

Caffeine

Caffeine, in the form of coffee, tea, and soda, does not usually cause a problem for breastfeeding babies. Some experts recommend limiting daily coffee intake to less than 25 oz (about 750 mL)—a little more than two 10-oz cups of coffee per day.

Rest

A breastfeeding parent needs rest to recover after childbirth, cope with stress, and make milk. Finding time for a daily rest period is helpful. When things get busy, remembering to set aside time during the day to rest may require a special note or phone reminder. It's important to avoid answering emails, text messages, or phone calls during rest time.

Talk to your lactation specialist about the need to wake up once or twice during the night to pump and express breast milk. Failing to pump at night is one of the most common reasons for low milk supply.

Prescription Medications, Over-the-Counter Medications, and Herbs

Breastfeeding parents need to tell the NICU team about every prescription medication, every over-the-counter medication (for example, cold remedies, antacids), and any herbs or supplements they take. A few of these, such as medications containing codeine, can be unsafe during breastfeeding. As a rule, breastfeeding parents should ask their baby's care providers before taking any medication, herb, or nutritional supplement while providing breast milk for their baby.

Alcohol

Many parents have questions about drinking alcohol once pregnancy is over. Possible long-term effects of alcohol in breast milk remain unknown, especially in preterm babies whose brains are still developing. Because alcohol passes into breast milk, and there is no known safe amount of alcohol exposure for babies, health professionals advise breastfeeding people to avoid consuming alcohol while providing breast milk. If a breastfeeding parent has an occasional alcoholic beverage, it should be limited to a single standard drink right after nursing or pumping milk, and breastfeeding or pumping should be avoided for 2 hours after the drink.

Tobacco and Marijuana

Nicotine and other poisons in cigarettes pass into breast milk and into your baby. You may have been able to stop smoking during pregnancy, but many parents start again during the NICU stay. Cigarettes expose your baby to secondhand and thirdhand smoke and increase your baby's risk of sudden infant death syndrome (SIDS). Breastfeeding parents who smoke should breastfeed their baby before they smoke. Some methods used to stop smoking (patches, gum, and some medications) can be used safely while breastfeeding. Get help and advice to stop smoking while your baby is in the NICU.

Marijuana is now legal in many states; however, this does not mean it is safe to use during breastfeeding. Tetrahydrocannabinol (THC) is the main chemical compound in marijuana and has been found in the stool (poop) of babies whose parents smoke marijuana, which means THC is absorbed and metabolized by the baby. Tetrahydrocannabinol has been found in levels up to 8 times higher in a parent's breast milk than in their bloodstream. Marijuana passes rapidly to the baby's brain and is also stored for weeks in the baby's fatty tissue. At this time, there is no strong research to evaluate the effects of marijuana on baby brain development, but there is some evidence that exposure to marijuana during critical periods of brain development can affect a child's learning abilities and emotional behaviors. In addition, exposure to secondhand marijuana smoke is associated with risk of SIDS, even though breastfeeding reduces the risk of SIDS. Because marijuana passes into breast milk, consider abstaining from marijuana use, especially while your preterm baby's brain is still developing.

Cocaine, Heroin, Amphetamines, Ecstasy, Designer Drugs, and Other Harmful Substances

It is important for breastfeeding parents to tell their NICU team if they use drugs or other potentially harmful substances. These pass through the parent's breast milk to their baby and sometimes produce tragic side effects. Your NICU team can tell you how long after using these substances you should delay breastfeeding or whether you should "pump and dump" your breast milk. Your health care professionals can be an advocate and provide referrals to helpful resources. Your well-being and the health of your baby are their top priorities. Let your team help find assistance so you can be the best parents possible.

Breastfeeding Challenges

Breastfeeding can be especially challenging for parents and babies in the NICU. In the beginning, it may seem like you are participating in the feeding process and your baby is not. This is normal. Give yourself and your baby time to learn, and ask for help when you encounter problems.

Babies Who Cannot Latch On

A few conditions make it difficult or nearly impossible for a baby to latch on. Babies with abnormal openings (*clefts*) in the roof of their mouth (*palate*) or abnormalities of the gum or jawbone may have difficulty latching on and creating suction. Some babies with nervous system or heart abnormalities will not have enough strength or coordination to suck effectively. If your baby has one of these problems, talk with your NICU team.

Nipple Preference

Because bottle-feeding is frequently a component of a baby's nutrition plan in the NICU, parents and staff worry about *nipple preference* or *nipple confusion*. This describes a situation in which a baby develops difficulty with breastfeeding after exposure to bottles. To avoid giving bottles to breastfeeding babies, some nurseries use techniques such as finger feeding or cup feeding. With finger feeding, the baby sucks on a gloved finger and a thin feeding tube is slipped into the baby's mouth. With cup feeding, the baby is held upright and small amounts of milk are placed on the baby's tongue with a cup or spoon. These methods have been researched and they do, to some extent, enhance breastfeeding success.

If breastfeeding has been going well for a few days, supplementing breastfeeding with bottle-feeding does not usually interfere with breastfeeding success. If you notice that breastfeeding is not going as well after exposure to bottle-feeding, talk with your NICU team and discuss the various options.

> " To treat her chronic kidney disease, they increased Meridith's fluid intake and calories, which meant she was never hungry, so despite our best efforts and a lot of help from her care team, Meridith just wasn't interested in breastfeeding. Even though I couldn't feed her directly from the source, I was able to pump for her for almost 3 years. "
>
> *Mary Ellen, mother of* **Meridith**

Decreasing Milk Supply

After the second or third week of pumping, some breastfeeding parents notice they are producing less milk. This is less likely to happen if they have a hospital-quality electric pump in good working order, use the double-pumping kit, use breast massage before or during pumping, and are pumping at least 8 times a day. If parents skip a pumping session and let their breasts become overly full, their milk supply will decrease. Pumping frequency is important. Short, frequent pumping (10 minutes, 10 times per day) is better than pumping longer but less often (20 minutes, 5 times per day).

On the other hand, some breastfeeding parents who pump frequently still have trouble making enough milk and become frustrated when told to pump more often. Feeling anxious or exhausted, not eating or drinking enough, becoming ill, or taking some medications can decrease a parent's milk supply. Stress reduction and spending more skin-to-skin time with the baby may increase supply. Consider low milk supply a signal that additional rest and supportive care may be needed.

Skin-to-skin care is not only good for **Meridith;** it can help increase her mom's milk supply.

Although some recommend various medications or herbal supplements to improve milk supply, there is little scientific evidence regarding their safety or efficacy. If you are considering trying one of these methods to increase milk supply, seek advice from your lactation specialist and approach this as a team decision.

Too Much Breast Milk

Sometimes, a breastfeeding parent will produce so much milk, they are able to donate it to help other babies. On a much sadder note, a person who loses their baby may also consider donating their milk. Ask your lactation specialist if there is a milk bank donation center near your home or the hospital. The person donating the milk will undergo a few blood tests to make sure they do not have any diseases that could harm another person's baby. Your gift of breast milk can make a big difference in the life of someone else's NICU baby.

If You Can't Provide Breast Milk

Families feed formula to their babies in the NICU for many different reasons. Sometimes, a parent tries and is unable to produce enough milk, or the baby is unable to breastfeed. Sometimes, medical problems make breastfeeding impossible. Unless there is a medical reason for not breastfeeding, the NICU team will probably encourage you to provide milk or consider using donor breast milk. Consider the pros and cons carefully and make the choice that is right for you and your baby. The NICU staff will support your decision and encourage your active participation in feeding your new baby.

Breast Problems

Sore Nipples

If your nipples become sore from pumping, try turning the pump's suction down, temporarily limiting pumping time to no more than 10 minutes, and applying modified lanolin around the areola before pumping. In addition, you may use a soft, flexible insert made for the electric pump that helps take the pressure off of your sore spot.

Yeast Infection (Thrush)

If your nipples suddenly become sore after being pain-free, or if your nipple pain is not associated with feeding or pumping, you may have a yeast infection. Babies often develop an oral yeast infection, called *thrush,* which appears as a milky white coating on the tongue and inner cheeks. Thrush is particularly common in babies who have received antibiotics. Breastfeeding may cause people to develop very sore nipples—which may look perfectly normal or be quite pink—as well as burning, shooting, or stabbing pains in the breasts. Check your baby's mouth periodically for signs of thrush on the tongue and roof of the mouth.

To treat the yeast infection, you and your baby must be treated together, at the same time. You will need a cream for your nipples, and your baby will receive a liquid medication. During the treatment, you and your baby's caregivers must sterilize pacifiers, breast pump parts, bottle nipples, and anything else that might reinfect your baby's mouth and your breasts. You can continue to breastfeed during treatment. For some breastfeeding parents, topical treatment alone will not suffice and they will need a 2- to 3-week course of an oral antifungal medication. This medicine is safe to take while breastfeeding or expressing milk for a preterm baby.

Mastitis

If you develop fever and chills, along with a hot, red, tender area on your breast, you probably have a breast infection called *mastitis*. Most cases of mastitis require 2 to 3 weeks of antibiotic treatment. Under ordinary circumstances, parents with mastitis who have healthy full-term babies should continue to breastfeed or pump because the germ is probably in the baby's mouth already. In the NICU, if your baby has not yet nursed at your breast, your baby's neonatologist may want to discuss the risks and benefits of feeding your breast milk to your baby while you have mastitis. If you are advised to discard your breast milk while you have mastitis, continue to pump your breasts ("pump and dump") so you can resume breastfeeding as soon as the infection clears up.

Clogged Ducts

A clogged duct produces a red, hot, tender lump on one breast that improves or goes away within about 2 to 3 days. Unlike mastitis, there is no fever. However, if left untreated, it could progress to mastitis.

Treat this problem as if you were coming down with a cold: Take it easy for a couple of days, get enough sleep, and drink extra fluids. In addition, soak your breast several times a day in a tub of warm water, massage it gently (squeezing is painful and not helpful), and pump more frequently. Sometimes, as the clog moves down the duct, a painful white spot develops on the tip of the nipple. This will go away after the clogged duct is clear again.

Clogged ducts are sometimes caused by a mechanical obstruction—for example, an underwire bra that presses on the breast, a shoulder strap, or your sleep position. Talk to a lactation specialist if you get clogged ducts often.

If You Need to Stop Breastfeeding

Even under the best of circumstances, not all parents and babies can breastfeed. It's normal to grieve the loss of something you looked forward to and valued. If you pumped for even a few days, you truly did breastfeed. Your baby will experience some long-lasting health benefits from receiving even a little of your milk. If possible, consider donor breast milk for your baby. Your lactation specialist and NICU team can advise you about this.

If you can stop breastfeeding over a period of days or a few weeks, your milk supply will gradually diminish and cause little discomfort. But if you have an abundant milk supply and stop breastfeeding suddenly, you may be very uncomfortable. If you experience painfully full breasts when you stop breastfeeding, read the section below titled If You Experience Breast Engorgement.

If You Experience Breast Engorgement

After you give birth, your body produces hormones that signal your breasts to make milk. In 2 to 3 days, your breasts swell with milk. If you don't remove the milk by nursing your baby or pumping, your breasts may become rock-hard and painful. The swelling may extend into your armpits, making even simple movements uncomfortable. You may develop a mild fever. This combination of symptoms is called *engorgement*.

After 2 or 3 days of engorgement, you'll notice your breasts are softer and more comfortable. If you are not breastfeeding, they will return to their pre-pregnancy size in several weeks. Until then, you may notice milk leaking from the nipples. Some people who do not breastfeed

---

Managing Breast Engorgement

While you wait for the engorgement to resolve naturally, try these comfort measures.

- If you do not plan to breastfeed, use a breast pump or hand express just enough milk to relieve the pressure. You can discard the milk or ask the hospital staff for containers so it can be given to your baby for these few days. As the swelling subsides, gradually pump or express less often. In a few days, you'll be able to stop altogether.

- Apply cold compresses, such as gel packs made for this purpose, a bag of frozen peas, wet washcloths chilled in the freezer, or the classic Australian remedy of cold raw cabbage leaves.

- Wear a bra if it fits well and feels good. If you have a sports bra, try that. Wear it to bed if the pain is keeping you awake at night.

- Take a pain reliever recommended by your health care professional.

- Try heat to relieve the pain. Wrap your breasts in warm, wet washcloths (covered with plastic wrap to keep the heat in), or take a warm shower, allowing any milk produced to flow down the drain.

(or stop breastfeeding) notice leaking for several months. This is normal, but leaking can be prolonged by anything that causes nipple stimulation—for example, running or other exercise that causes your breasts to bounce and any stimulation that involves your breasts and nipples. If you still have milk 6 to 12 months after giving birth, or if you think the leaking is excessive (and you've tried reducing the amount of nipple stimulation), talk to your health care professional.

Bottle-feeding Basics for All NICU Babies

Most preterm babies will get some of their nutrition from bottle-feeding. You may also hear this called "nipple feeding." Even preterm babies who are learning to breastfeed will likely get some breast milk from a bottle, so parents who are providing breast milk also need to know the basics of how to feed their baby from a bottle.

Bottles and Nipples

Bottles designed for babies in the NICU usually hold 1½ or 2 oz, and measurements are marked on the side of the bottle. The NICU staff measure the amount by using the more accurate metric system and will describe it in milliliters. One ounce is about 30 mL. A very preterm newborn's first feeding is usually only 1 to 2 mL (about ¼ teaspoon). Larger preterm newborns may begin feedings with 10 to 20 mL (⅓ to ⅔ oz).

The nipples for bottles come in a variety of shapes and sizes. Some nipples are smaller and softer, while others are larger and stiffer. The NICU staff will help determine which nipples work best for your baby.

Learning to Bottle-feed

Feeding a baby in the NICU can be challenging. Here are some tips for bottle-feeding your newborn in the NICU. Additional tips for feeding at home are discussed in Chapter 9.

Watch Your Baby's Feeding Cues

Do what you can to help your baby be alert and ready when you offer the bottle. If you notice preparations for feeding (for example, diapering, dressing) seem to tire your baby, feed first and delay diapering until later. Although some parents prefer to warm formula before feeding, most babies accept room-temperature formula just fine. When feeding breast milk, the NICU staff will teach you the correct way to warm breast milk from the refrigerator or freezer.

Eliana practices bottle-feeding with her dad.

Position Your Baby Properly

Hold your baby comfortably in your arms, close to your body, with the baby's head slightly raised. If your baby's arms and legs are limp, bend them into a flexed position. Some babies will feed better when lying on their side. The NICU staff will help identify the best position for your baby. Don't sit where bright lights will shine in your baby's face, and take a break if the noise in the NICU becomes too loud. Never prop the bottle because the baby could choke and breathe it back into the lungs (*aspirate*).

A preterm baby may try to bottle-feed with their tongue on top of the nipple. You can help position the nipple correctly by guiding the nipple, with your finger on top of it, into the mouth.

Let Your Baby Set the Pace

Relax, and let your baby set the pace during bottle-feeding. Don't try to hurry the process by wiggling, turning, and pumping the nipple in your baby's mouth. Forcing milk into a baby's mouth can cause choking, breathing pauses (*apnea*), slow heart rate (*bradycardia*), and *oxygen desaturation*.

On the other hand, a feeding that lasts longer than about 30 minutes may leave your baby exhausted. Often, a baby who successfully finishes part of the feeding will receive the remainder through the feeding tube. You will learn to read your baby's cues and decide whether it's time to stop feeding or to continue. This partnership with your baby—this mutual understanding— takes time, but soon you will become the expert at feeding your baby.

Skin-to-Skin (Kangaroo) Care

If you are bottle-feeding your baby, ask your baby's nurse about skin-to-skin (kangaroo) care (see Chapter 6). This method of skin-to-skin holding is not just for breastfeeding parents. Both parents can enjoy the skin-to-skin warmth of kangaroo care, and parents appreciate the family closeness it offers. Providing skin-to-skin time with your baby in the NICU is helpful for bonding and establishing caregiving confidence. After you take your baby home, continue to find time to enjoy the pleasure of skin-to-skin contact—for example, after a bath or first thing in the morning.

Your Baby Needs You

Feeding is a common area of concern for the families of full-term and preterm babies, for parents of babies who are healthy at birth, and for those whose babies need intensive care. Not only is nourishment vital to your baby's well-being, but feeding is closely related to many other areas of your baby's care and healthy future. Whatever your concerns, questions, or struggles, specialists in the NICU will help you find the right answers.

Abel

Born at 22 weeks, 5 days

Abel was born at 22 weeks, 5 days in fall of 2021. He weighed 1 pound 8 ounces. He was in the NICU for 207 days (about 7 months). Abel is the first 22-week survivor in our hospital's NICU.

We have 3 other children, who are now 11, 6, and 2 years old. All were born preterm, but the earliest birth was 33½ weeks of gestation. My pregnancy with Abel was high risk from the beginning. Aside from my diabetes, I had placenta accreta (when blood vessels and parts of the placenta grow into the uterine wall) and a velamentous cord insertion (when the umbilical cord attaches to the membranes surrounding the placenta instead of inserting into the placenta). Both of these rare complications increase the risk of bleeding and can affect the baby's growth and nutrition. I was very closely monitored with weekly ultrasounds and was doing okay.

One evening, I suddenly felt faint and got sick. I had intense burning abdominal pain. I was bleeding out, and paramedics raced me to the closest hospital in our neighborhood. After consulting with my OB team in the city, they took me to surgery. Abel was not expected to live; the goal was to save my life. My uterus had spontaneously ruptured, and I also had a bowel perforation. Abel was delivered alive and MedFlight took him to a NICU in the city. I received 20 units of blood and was transferred to the ICU. Two days later, I woke up intubated and learned I had a son.

On day 5, I was transported to the same hospital as Abel's, but I was too unstable to see him until the evening of day 7. The nurses encouraged me to visit him, but I was afraid.

I didn't know what to expect or if such a premature baby would even look like a baby. Finally, I worked up the nerve to see him and discovered he was beautiful. Just very very tiny.

At that time, my husband had not yet told me about Abel's first infection because he didn't want to upset me, but Abel had been diagnosed with *aspergillosis*. That's an unusual (and often fatal) fungal infection that attacks the respiratory system. There is not much research on how to treat this in preemies and most babies die.

Abel's mother spent several days in the ICU after Abel's birth.

Abel was born at 22 weeks, 5 days, gestation.

Abel was on medication for 4 months and beat it. That was the first of many infection scares for Abel.

It was really hard to involve any of our family in the NICU experience because of COVID and no NICU visitors were allowed. We used FaceTime a lot and took many pictures. Our parents met Abel a few times during his most critical moments in the beginning, and then not again until right before discharge. During Abel's second week, the doctors thought he was not going to make it through the night, so they let our 2 daughters come in to say goodbye. That was the only time they got to see him in the NICU. Our youngest child, Jack, met Abel a week before we brought Abel home.

Abel experienced most of the usual problems of an extremely premature birth. He was intubated for 110 days and has chronic lung disease. He is still on oxygen via nasal cannula, and his oxygen needs are assessed and adjusted every week. Some weeks he needs more oxygen, sometimes less. He had heart surgery to ligate his patent ductus arteriosus (PDA). He had retinopathy of prematurity (ROP) but amazingly that has resolved.

Feeding him has been difficult. He did not start on tube feeds until he was 2 months old. I was still pumping for my 9-month old, so I was able to pump milk to supply the small drops they put into his mouth for immunotherapy. He easily aspirates, so he eventually got a gastrostomy tube (G-tube). Currently, he gets his G-tube feeding every 3 hours, takes 5 to 10 mL of breast milk in a bottle several times a day for practice, and can practice breastfeeding after I pump. Eventually, he will take his feeds by mouth.

I was in the NICU every day for most of Abel's stay. I learned a lot about Abel by spending time with him. I learned what made him happy. I learned his distress signals and didn't even need to look at the monitors to know when something was wrong. That helped me prepare for his discharge, and I was really excited about bringing my baby home. I was also very scared that I wouldn't be able to take great care of him and would possibly

Abel enjoys his first tub bath at age 3 months.

mess up on things such as medications. I was taking him from the only home he had ever known and people who were with him daily. I worried that we were not going to have a strong bond. All of those worries faded over time. I quickly found out that I am capable of taking care of my son. Our connection is very strong and has grown stronger since spending quality time with each other at home. That has been a big thing for me, especially mentally.

Abel had a great NICU team. We got to know a lot of doctors who rotated in and out of the NICU, but it's so important to forge relationships with the nurse practitioners and the nurses who are there for the long haul. The consistency was there, and month after month getting to know them and how they care for and know my son made a world of difference. We are still in touch with all of them and they come to see him often. Our NICU social worker was my rock (and still is) and I don't know what I would have done without her. All these important people, including the front desk employees who talk to you every day, become a part of your family.

I'm looking forward to Abel's future. I have so much joy in knowing that Abel even has a future. I look forward to doing all the things with him that I was able to do with our other children. I look forward to him crushing his milestones his way and in his own time. He is truly a miracle and every day that I have with him is such a blessing.

Shana, mother of Abel

Abel enjoys socializing and has a great smile. His G-tube for feeding is visible on his abdomen.

Sienna

Born at 31 weeks, 4 days

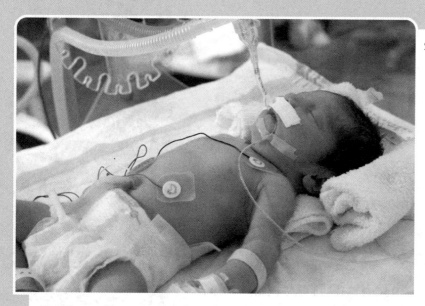

Sienna soon after birth.

Sienna was born at 31 weeks 4 days of gestation, after a placental abruption caused her premature birth. She spent her first 19 days in the NICU, learning to breathe and eat on her own. I lived about 45 minutes away from the hospital, so every day I drove there, spent the day, and tearfully departed for home in the late hours of the evening. In the beginning, I knew it was necessary, and Sienna had to be under their care and supervision.

The doctors and nurses provided incredible care for her in those early, fragile days, and for that I could not possibly be more grateful. Sienna proved, very early on, that she was a fighter and did not plan to stay there for too long. Within a few days, she was breathing on her own and out of the incubator. She spent the majority of her stay learning how to eat on her own, without a feeding tube. Every day, Sienna progressed little by little.

Sienna making progress.

When she was finally able to come home, my heart was full of happiness but also anxiety, as she would no longer be hooked up to sensors that would alarm to tell me something was off. Thankfully, the transition from NICU to home was seamless.

Today, Sienna is 6 years old. She has no health problems and no development issues. She is incredibly smart and one of the strongest readers in her class. She was blessed with artistic talent, as well as a great left-handed shot with her bow and arrow. She has a beautiful, giving, and compassionate heart to go along with her resilient "tough girl" attitude. I believe that Sienna's entrance into this world was one that was predestined in order to shape her into the sweet, smart, and healthy little girl that she is today. She makes my heart soar and has given me purpose in life. **Read more about Sienna in "Where Are They Now?" in the Appendix.**

"Sienna at 5 years old in this photo. She loves to be outside! This was her first time catching a frog. She is fearless and brave."

Kaitlynn, mother of Sienna

Kaitlynn, mother of Sienna

Sienna, at age 6 years.

CHAPTER 8

Homeward Bound

> " We took Ethan to the hospital
> to see his new brother and sister.
> He was happy to see them, but he had
> a big meltdown when we told him both
> babies were coming home soon.
> 'I asked for a sister,' he said,
> 'so we only take my sister home.'
>
> *Parina, mother of **Isaac** and **Eliza*** "

As your baby grows and the most serious medical problems begin to resolve, you will start thinking about getting ready to bring your baby home. During this phase of the hospital stay, there is generally a greater focus on parental involvement. Learning to care for your baby becomes the focal point of your time.

The Intermediate Care Experience

Some babies go home directly from the neonatal intensive care unit (NICU), but some are moved to a less intensive environment, sometimes called *intermediate care, NICU step-down, special care, feeding-and-growing, or Level II unit.* One day, your NICU team may tell you, "It's graduation day! Your baby is leaving the NICU and moving to the intermediate care nursery. It won't be long until you can take your baby home."

Graduation sounds like progress (and it is!), but what else changes? Being a NICU parent has meant dealing with daily changes, but by now you have developed a comfort level with the NICU staff, equipment, routines, and procedures. Things may be different in the new unit. This change means another period of adjustment.

The new unit may be within the NICU itself or nearby. Some NICUs transfer babies to a community hospital closer to home and, maybe, where your NICU journey first began. Knowing what to expect in the way of routines, staff members, and your role during this period will help you feel more comfortable and learn what you'll need to know when your baby comes home.

Transferring to Intermediate Care

With few exceptions, your transfer out of intensive care means that your baby is past the major medical problems and is on the road home.

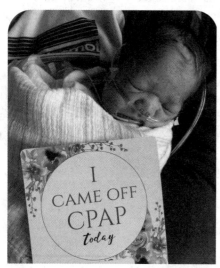

Eliana's graduation from CPAP to nasal cannula is a significant step toward hospital discharge.

Often, the intermediate care setting is quieter, less hectic, and a better place to establish sleep/wake cycles. Because growing babies need a lot of undisturbed rest, feeding time is often the best time for interaction; therefore, your team may suggest you spend this time learning about your baby's emerging personality, cues, and behaviors.

Your baby no longer requires frequent intensive nursing care, so expect your baby's nurse to be caring for 2 to 3 other babies. Depending on the hospital, the nursing staff in the intermediate care setting may be the same as the staff in the NICU, and you may even have the same primary nurse. In many hospitals, your baby's doctors and consulting specialists will remain the same in the new setting. Occupational or physical therapists may work with you and your baby more frequently now on feeding skills, positioning, comforting, and other behavioral and physical tasks.

Transferring to a Community Hospital

If your baby was transferred to the NICU from another hospital, your NICU team may discuss returning to your community hospital for continued convalescence and preparation for discharge. *Back transport*—also called *return transport*—is common in hospitals where NICU beds are used for the sickest babies and less intensive care is done in community hospital special care nurseries. The community hospital is often closer to your home and may allow you to spend more quality time with your baby.

Community hospitals with special care nurseries are pleased and excited to care for your baby. You may discover that you can learn to care for your baby in a more relaxed setting and also receive more individual attention. People who can help you and your baby make the transition to home are available at the community hospital and are familiar with local support sources, such as medical equipment supply companies and community home health services. If your baby requires complex care, you can ask the community nursery about its access to specialty staff—such as neurologists, ophthalmologists, and pulmonologists—for consultations.

Becoming Comfortable in New Surroundings

If your baby moves to an intermediate care nursery or community hospital that has a different staff, you may miss the comfortable working relationships you shared with the NICU staff. You and your baby may need some time to get acquainted with a new team and learn how to communicate well with that team. Eventually, you will develop trusting relationships with staff members in the intermediate care nursery, just as you did with those in the NICU.

You may need to adjust to new routines and procedures. One of the biggest challenges of becoming comfortable in a new setting is understanding that *different* is not necessarily *wrong*. In addition to learning about the new unit routines, communicate your baby's likes and dislikes, including your baby's typical behavior patterns, with the staff. They will be most appreciative of the information during this period when everyone is getting acquainted.

Emotional Changes

As things slow down, you may find that emotions from the past weeks are catching up with you. You may have been too frightened or overwhelmed to express some of those feelings, but now they seem to come tumbling out at your partner, the nursery staff, and anyone else who is willing to listen. This is common and will subside eventually.

If your anxiety does not decrease, or if you are having trouble sleeping, eating, or taking care of your daily needs, tell your doctor or your baby's social worker or nurse. They can help you find resources before your baby is ready to come home.

> My advice to NICU parents would be to advocate not only for your baby, but for yourself. If you suffer from anxiety that doesn't go away or interferes with your daily life or your ability to be the parent you want to be, tell someone and get help. The sooner you get help, the sooner you'll be on your way to recovery.
>
> *Alex, father of **Pascal***

Adjusting to the Change

The transfer process is a lot of activity for a preterm baby. You may find that your baby is sleepier than usual or may not tolerate feedings well for the first 24 hours in the new environment. Some babies require a slight increase in supplemental oxygen following a transport, or they might lose a bit of weight for the first few days. Given an opportunity for quiet rest, your baby will quickly recover and adapt to this new setting.

Preparing for discharge can be almost as stressful as your first days in the NICU. Matthew spends some relaxing quiet time with twins **Bailey Jo** and **Abraham** as discharge day approaches.

Your Expanding Role in Care

During this phase of the hospital stay, you and your baby will master the skills necessary for discharge. This is the time to take a more active role in your baby's care.

As discharge nears, you'll need the nurse's help less often. Your baby's nurse may still talk you through more complex tasks, but by now you should be fairly comfortable taking a temperature or changing a diaper. Use your nurse as a resource whenever you have questions or need assistance during this learning period.

> ❝ I learned a lot about **Abel** by spending time with him. I learned what made him happy. I learned his distress signals and didn't even need to look at the monitors to know when something was wrong. That helped me prepare for his discharge. ❞
>
> *Shana, mother of **Abel***

What Do You Need to Know?

You'll need to know your baby's schedule to participate in care. Ask about the feeding schedule, bath time, and special treatments, such as respiratory or physical therapy. Let the nurses know what you feel comfortable doing (for example, changing a diaper) and what skills you're ready to learn (such as giving medications). Nurses will gladly save a feeding or bath for parents or rearrange your baby's schedule to fit your schedule if this is discussed ahead of time. The intermediate care nursery also provides an excellent opportunity for parents to begin or continue skin-to-skin (kangaroo) care.

With many of his medical issues behind him, **Nathan** gains weight and improves his feeding skills in this phase of his NICU journey.

Hands-on Skills You Will Need Before Discharge

- Feeding
- Diapering
- Dressing
- Taking a temperature
- Bathing
- Giving medication
- How to use any medical devices your baby will need after discharge
- Infant cardiopulmonary resuscitation (CPR)

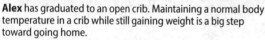

Alex has graduated to an open crib. Maintaining a normal body temperature in a crib while still gaining weight is a big step toward going home.

The NICU team encourages you to care for your baby as soon as you and the baby are ready. This mother is learning to bathe her baby.

Courtesy of University of Washington Medical Center, Seattle, WA.

Milestones a Preterm Baby Will Meet Before Discharge

Your baby will need to:

- "Outgrow" apneic events and periodic breathing that cause bradycardia and desaturation.
- Have a safe discharge feeding plan.
- Show a regular trend of weight gain on the discharge feeding plan.
- Maintain a normal body temperature in an open crib.

" I grew more confident as I got to know Lucy and her care team. Sometimes it may feel like you don't have a say in the process, but I learned we were Lucy's voice and needed to speak up even when we didn't know exactly what to say. "

*Kate, mother of **Lucy***

Common Health Issues During This Phase

Now that your baby is in the "feeding and growing" phase of care, you are past many of the serious problems that may have been present while your baby was critically ill. As your baby approaches hospital discharge, here are some common health issues that may still require attention.

Bronchopulmonary Dysplasia

Preterm babies who have *bronchopulmonary dysplasia* (also called *BPD* or *chronic lung disease*) may still require breathing support, additional oxygen, and medications. As oral feeding progresses, there may be days when your baby is not breathing as comfortably or needs more oxygen. These ups and downs are normal but can be very frustrating. During this phase of care, your medical team will determine if support can be weaned before hospital discharge or if your baby will still need some type of breathing support at home.

Apnea and Bradycardia

Apnea, bradycardia, and desaturations are a common problem for preterm babies, and these events may continue during this phase. Unless they are a side effect of another illness, these events go away as your baby's brain matures and most often resolve before your baby's original due date. Some babies, born extremely prematurely, may continue to have occasional apnea and bradycardia events for several weeks after their due date. The staff will monitor the frequency, intensity, and duration of the episodes. If medication is used to control apnea, it may be stopped before hospital discharge and your baby will be monitored for a period of time to ensure that the medication is no longer needed. Sometimes, waiting for apnea and bradycardia to resolve is the final step before a baby is ready for discharge.

Gastroesophageal Reflux

A condition known as *gastroesophageal reflux* (*GER*) occurs when swallowed milk moves back up the food pipe (*esophagus*). Gastroesophageal reflux is considered a normal physiologic process in newborns. Some babies with GER might spit up frequently and lose a lot of what was eaten. You may notice signs of discomfort during feeding and poor weight gain with frequent GER, which can be frustrating for parents and other caregivers. Some babies will experience improvement with frequent burping, adjusting the head of the bed, changing the baby's position during or after feeding, changing the timing or duration of the feeding, or changing the baby's formula if the baby is not receiving breast milk. There is no scientific evidence that any treatment significantly improves GER. Most preterm babies show at least occasional episodes of GER, and most will outgrow it as they reach their original due date. In some cases, reflux can be associated with severe symptoms or complications; such patients are referred to as having *gastroesophageal reflux disease* (*GERD*), and consultation with a gastrointestinal specialist may be needed to help resolve this problem.

Anemia

Growing preterm babies frequently have anemia of prematurity (low red blood cell [RBC] count). Recall that anemia of prematurity occurs because RBC production temporarily stops after birth (see Chapter 5). The number of RBCs, measured by the *hemoglobin level* or *hematocrit*, reaches its lowest value between 4 and 10 weeks after birth and gradually increases afterward.

If your baby still requires additional oxygen, the nursery team may recommend occasional blood transfusions. If your baby is in stable condition and growing well, the nursery team may allow the hemoglobin level to drop to stimulate the baby's own RBC production system. In addition, growing preterm babies may receive extra iron to support blood cell production. In some hospitals, an injected medication called *erythropoietin* (EPO) will be given to stimulate RBC production. If your baby still has anemia at the time of discharge, your pediatrician may continue to check the hemoglobin level until it starts to increase.

Hernias

Preterm babies are at risk for hernias—when a loop of intestine moves through a muscle weakness or other opening inside the body.

Inguinal Hernia

The most common hernia is called an *inguinal hernia*. This condition occurs most often in boys and usually presents as a bulge in the groin, especially after crying or straining during a bowel movement. Sometimes girls develop inguinal hernias, which cause a bulge, or swelling, above or along the outer labia (near the vaginal opening); hernias in girls can contain either intestine or an ovary, which sits near the site of the hernia.

A boy's testicles are inside the abdomen during development and stay high in the groin (*inguinal canal*) until about 32 weeks' gestation. At that time, the testicles descend through the canal into the scrotum. Although possible in all babies, preterm infants are at higher risk for a hernia, which occurs when part of the intestine also pushes through the canal into the scrotum. This may affect one or both sides and appears as a swelling above or in the scrotum. Sometimes the swelling is due to simple fluid buildup in a tiny channel that is too small to let intestine out; this is called a *hydrocele*, which is not dangerous and usually goes away on its own without surgery.

If the intestine can be easily and gently pushed back through the opening (the hernia is *reducible*), immediate surgical correction is not necessary. Surgery to repair the hernia may occur before discharge, or it may be delayed until your baby is older. If the intestine becomes trapped in the groin, labia, or scrotum (*incarcerated hernia*), the hernia and overlying skin will become swollen, discolored, and painful, and immediate surgery may be necessary if it cannot be reduced.

Umbilical Hernia

Hernias also commonly occur around the umbilical area or belly button. In this case, the ring of muscle and supporting tissue at the base of the belly button is loose and allows loops of intestine to push outward when the baby cries or strains. As long as there is no pain, redness, or discoloration, there is no cause for concern. A small *umbilical hernia* often corrects itself or becomes significantly smaller within 5 years as your baby grows and the abdominal muscles strengthen and thicken. In general, surgical correction is only recommended for umbilical hernias that become trapped (*incarcerated*), are painful, or have not completely closed by 5 years of age.

> 66 A stay in the NICU is going to be temporary. They won't let you stay there forever even on those days when it really feels like you will be there forever. While it is difficult to not constantly look for the finish line (and everyone will ask, 'When is the baby coming home?'), try to take it day by day and minute by minute and find happiness and joy in the experience. The NICU is an amazing place when you stop and look around. 99

*Kate, mother of **Lucy***

Deciding About Male Circumcision

Opinions vary about male *circumcision* (removal of the skin covering the tip of the penis). For some, male circumcision is a religious obligation, and for others it is a personal decision. The American Academy of Pediatrics (AAP) states that the health benefits of male circumcision outweigh the risks of the procedure, but the benefits are not great enough to recommend universal newborn circumcision. Specific benefits include prevention of urinary tract infections, penile cancer, and transmission of some sexually transmitted infections, including HIV. Risks of the procedure include bleeding, incomplete circumcision requiring revision surgery, and injury to the penis.

In most circumstances, the decision regarding male circumcision is up to the parents, in the context of their religious, ethical, and cultural beliefs. If you decide that male circumcision is the right choice, check with your baby's care team to discuss timing of the procedure and with your insurance carrier to see if the procedure is covered.

Predischarge Testing

While you're learning all you can about your baby's care, the health care team is planning your baby's final tests and preparing for discharge. Common discharge tests are explained here, but not all babies require all the tests discussed, and some may need more. Ask your baby's team what to expect as discharge draws near.

Eye Examination

If your baby was 30 weeks' gestation or less or weighed 1,500 g (3 lb 5 oz) or less at birth, an eye examination performed by an ophthalmologist will be scheduled between 4 and 9 weeks of age. Babies born after 30 weeks' gestation and weighing between 1,500 and 2,000 g (3 lb 5 oz to 4 lb 6½ oz) may also have this type of eye examination if they were particularly sick in the newborn period. In some units, an ophthalmologist is not available to come to the hospital; in such cases, the nursery team will take photographs of your baby's eyes with a special digital camera and send them to a consulting ophthalmologist for evaluation. Follow-up examinations will be scheduled if necessary. The examination is to identify any changes in the sensitive tissue at the back of the eye caused by retinopathy of prematurity (see Chapter 5).

Hearing Test

Using electronic sound and response monitoring, automated hearing tests—also called *audiology screenings*—are used to help determine if your baby hears normally. Environmental conditions, such as surrounding noise or a crying baby, can cause inconclusive results. If this happens, a repeat test will be planned when your baby is sleeping and the room is quieter. After discharge, your child's hearing should be monitored by your pediatrician at periodic health examinations. If you are concerned about your baby's hearing, alert your pediatrician so additional testing can be scheduled if necessary.

> " Pascal weaned off his high-flow nasal cannula, finished his antibiotics, and then failed his car seat test, then again, then again. You know those 5 stages of grief? I was stuck oscillating between acceptance and bargaining: If he's not safe to go home, then we'll stay, of course we'll stay. But we don't live very far! I can get a different stroller that doesn't take the car seat! The kind with the bassinet! I won't leave him in bouncy seats! Each time, the nurse or the fellow would talk me through it: 'He's not safe to go home. He just needs more time.' "
>
> *Alex, father of **Pascal***

Car Safety Seats and the Car Safety Seat Test

After discharge, using an approved and well-fitting car safety seat every time your baby is in the car is one of the most important things you can do to protect your baby's health and safety. In all 50 states, car safety seat use is mandated by law. Each year, thousands of infants and young children are killed or injured in car crashes. Your lap is never a safe place for your baby in a moving vehicle.

All babies need to use a car safety seat that fits their weight, height, and any special needs. If your baby weighs less than 5 lb, check to see if the seat's manufacturer allows it to be used for babies at your child's weight. Some seats come with an additional insert that helps very small babies fit better, but parents should only use inserts that come in the box with the seat and never use any other product inside the car safety seat.

Ask your health care team if your baby will have a *car safety seat test* (sometimes called an *angle tolerance test*) before discharge. The AAP recommends this evaluation if your baby is born preterm or has certain other medical problems. During a car safety seat test, your baby is positioned in the car seat you bought and the baby's heart rate, breathing, and oxygen saturation are monitored for a period of time. The car safety seat test helps to determine if your baby can tolerate the upright position of the seat without having breathing problems. If your baby has apnea, bradycardia, or desaturations in the car seat, the team may suggest a different type of car safety seat that allows the baby to lie flat while traveling (*car bed*), investigate if there are other problems causing these events during the car seat test, or delay discharge to allow your baby additional time to grow before attempting the test again.

Nathan has passed his car safety seat test and his parents can feel more confident that he can tolerate this position in a car seat, an infant carrier, a baby seat, or a swing without bradycardia or desaturation.

Most car safety seats are not installed correctly in the car. If your hospital does not have a certified Child Passenger Safety technician on staff who can help you, you can find a certified technician at **http://cert.safekids.org** or by calling the National Highway Traffic Safety Administration Vehicle Safety Hotline at 888/327-4236. This should be done before your baby is discharged from the hospital so you can ensure that the car safety seat is correctly installed. To keep current on this topic, visit the official AAP website for parents at **www.HealthyChildren.org/carseat**.

Please use this QR code to go directly to http://cert.safekids.org.

Please use this QR code to go directly to www.HealthyChildren.org/carseat.

Pulse Oximetry Screen for Critical Congenital Heart Defects

All newborns are screened for *critical congenital heart disease* (CCHD) before they are discharged from the hospital nursery. Critical congenital heart diseases are life-threatening and not always diagnosed before birth or in the first few days after birth. The screening does not detect all forms of CCHD, but it is considered a valuable detection tool because an apparently healthy newborn who goes home with an undetected CCHD may be critically ill by the time parents notice signs of trouble and get the baby to an emergency department.

This screening measures blood oxygen saturation by placing a pulse oximeter on your baby's right hand and on either foot. An infant passes screening (a negative screen) if the oxygen saturation is 95 percent or greater in the right hand and foot and the difference is three points or less between the right hand and foot. If the baby "fails" the screening, it does not mean the baby has a heart defect, but the baby should be evaluated further, including having an echocardiogram before discharge.

The AAP recommends pulse oximetry screening for CCHD prior to discharge for any baby who has not already had an echocardiogram performed during their hospital stay. Because NICU babies may have been monitored with pulse oximetry numerous times and may have had other cardiac exams during their NICU stay, the pulse oximetry screen for critical congenital heart defects may not be necessary. Your team can discuss this with you. If the screen is still necessary, your team may delay the pulse oximetry screening test until your baby has been weaned from supplemental oxygen.

Immunizations

If your baby is in the hospital for 60 days or more, the medical team will talk to you about the immunizations routinely given at that time. These are the same vaccines your baby would receive in the doctor's office at a 2-month checkup and are important for your baby's health.

Immunizations for Your Baby

With few exceptions, the immunization schedule for preterm infants is the same as that for term infants. You don't have to correct for how early your baby was born. The first dose of hepatitis vaccine that is usually given right after birth may have been delayed, and your baby may need to "catch up." In addition, the rotavirus vaccine is a live virus vaccine; it may not be given until your baby is ready to leave the hospital, or it may be given in your pediatrician's office.

If your infant was very preterm or has significant heart disease, there is an increased risk of rehospitalization due to *respiratory syncytial virus* (*RSV*) infection. Your doctor will determine if your baby should receive a medication that can decrease this risk. This medication, called palivizumab (brand name Synagis), is given as an injection once a month for 1 to 5 months during the winter.

> "At a certain point, after another car seat test failure, his nurse decided we would do something fun, and she set up everything we needed for a bath and instructed me in how to wash him. I did not actually know how to bathe a baby, and to this day, I remain grateful for her teaching and for the photo she took of me bathing him. As a solo parent, it's remarkably hard to get photos of you and the baby together that's not a selfie, and as great as selfies are, there's something sweet about having both my hands in the photo, cradling him in the sink."

Alex, father of **Pascal**

> 66 John and I are so excited about getting our babies home, but also very nervous. They are going to be very susceptible to colds and other sickness, so we need to be diligent about keeping them as protected as possible. As much as we love company (and all our family and friends), we probably won't be able to see much of anybody. We will be pretty much homebound for much of the winter. We look forward to more visitors this spring! 99

Billie, mother of **Holland** *and* **Eden**

Immunizations for Parents and Family

Immunizing your baby is an important investment in health and protects your baby from rehospitalization, but your new baby is not the only one who needs immunizations. Be sure your other children and the adults in your home are up to date on all of their immunizations. Follow current guidance on COVID vaccination. Ask whether you or other family members need a whooping cough (*pertussis*) booster immunization. Everyone older than 6 months in your family, and everyone who will take care of your baby, should also receive the influenza vaccine before flu season starts each year. By immunizing yourself, your family, and your baby's caregivers, you are doing your best to protect your baby from preventable and potentially serious infections.

Getting What Your Baby Will Need

While your baby is growing stronger and getting ready to go home, it's time to pull out all the baby care books that you hid away because they seemed so irrelevant to your NICU experience. Review the baby supply and home preparation lists and start getting what you'll need. Now may also be the time to cue eager friends or family members who have been waiting for the right moment to give you a baby shower.

Shop Wisely

Some baby care items that sound like a good idea are totally unnecessary. For example, do not buy baby sleep positioners that are supposed to keep your baby correctly positioned for safe sleep. If your baby needs a positioner, it will be recommended by your baby's doctor or physical therapist. You do not need to buy extra pads or positioners to place in your baby's car safety seat. If it did not come with the seat, and if you did not use it during your baby's car safety seat test in the hospital, do not use it. Remember to ask your baby's health care team about any concerns you have regarding baby care items.

> " We started to see hope. We started our mission to bring our babies home. We did a deep cleaning of our home, prepped extra meals, and got 2 of everything for their arrival. "
>
> *Parina, mother of **Isaac** and **Eliza***

Clothing and Diapers

By the time they are ready for discharge, many preterm babies fit into newborn-sized clothes. You may decide to purchase a few "going out" items in preemie size for special occasions, but keep in mind that your baby will quickly outgrow them.

Newborn diapers generally work fine for most preterm babies at discharge. Some hospitals send a small supply of preemie diapers home with you. If necessary, you can buy extra-small diapers online or in many grocery stores and drugstores.

You may have a preference for cloth or disposable diapers. But as your baby grows, you may change your mind and decide to use a combination of cloth and disposable supplies.

Breastfeeding Aids

If you have been breastfeeding your baby, you will have the basic supplies already. Most breastfeeding parents of NICU graduates also need to continue to use a hospital-grade electric breast pump at home for a while after their baby's discharge.

What Does a Baby Need at Home?

Clothing
4 to 6 T-shirts
8 sleep gowns
6 one-piece T-shirts with snaps at waist
 or crotch
2 to 4 sweatshirts or sweaters
1 or 2 outfits for special occasions
6 pairs of booties or socks
12 fabric diaper covers if using cloth diapers
5 dozen cloth diapers (may also be used as
 burp cloths) or disposable diapers

Seasonal
Coat, knit hat
Cotton hat or bonnet

Bedtime
2 to 3 sleep sacks (no blankets in the crib)
2 to 4 tight-fitting crib sheets
2 waterproof mattress liners (goes under the
 crib sheet)
Nursery monitor (if you want to use one)
Nightlight

Bath Time
1 or 2 large, hooded towels
2 to 4 washcloths
Plastic bathtub
Foam bathtub liner (foam bath pillow)
Brush and comb set
Baby shampoo
Baby nail clippers

Health Care Supplies
Digital thermometer and lubricant
Infant acetaminophen as recommended by
 your baby's health care professional
Medicine syringe with accurate markings
Baby journal and calendar

Furniture
Bassinet or cradle (if baby's sleep location varies)
Crib and mattress or portable crib
Chest of drawers with anchors to prevent
 tip-overs and drawer latches/safety locks
Changing table with anchors to prevent
 tip-overs
Laundry hamper
Diaper pail for cloth diapers or garbage
 container

Outings
Diaper bag or backpack
Car safety seat
Stroller that is appropriate to your baby's needs

Breastfeeding
2 or 3 nursing bras
Nursing pads
Hospital-grade electric breast pump
Containers and labels for breast milk storage

Bottle-feeding
8 four-ounce or 8-ounce bottles and nipples
Bottle brush or dishwasher cage

Formula Feeding
Baby formula recommended by your baby's
 health care professional

Miscellaneous
2 or 3 pacifiers (if your baby uses one)
Baby toys and books
Baby memory book
Baby care books
Baby laundry soap

Later
Front carrier or backpack
Baby swing
High chair
Bibs
Feeding spoons and cups
Childproofing supplies

Breast Milk Supplements and Formula

Find out if your baby will be discharged with a breast milk supplement or preterm discharge formula. Ask your care team if there is a particular brand you need to purchase or if different brands are interchangeable. Locate the stores in your area that sell the supplement or formula you need. Large retail stores may stock preterm discharge formulas, but smaller stores may need to order them. If your baby requires a special formula, your local pharmacy may need to order it for you. Talk to your discharge planner, dietitian, or social worker to see if the supplement or formula you need is covered by insurance or the government-funded Women, Infants, and Children (WIC) program.

If you used a formula in the hospital, it was most likely provided in a ready-to-feed, premixed bottle. Ready-to-feed formula is convenient, but it is the most expensive. You may want to keep a couple of bottles of ready-to-feed formula in your diaper bag for emergencies during travel. After discharge, you may choose to buy formula as a liquid concentrate or powder that you mix with water. Talk to your care team about which type they recommend. Powder is the least expensive but has a greater risk of becoming contaminated with bacteria. In any case, make sure you carefully follow the instructions for mixing formula provided by your doctor and dietitian.

Water from most public water systems is acceptable for infant use. To be sure, however, ask your baby's care team about the necessity of boiling supplies when preparing formula, including the water used to dilute concentrate or powder formula. Most physicians are comfortable with a thorough washing of all supplies with hot soapy water and a bottle brush. Most dishwashers are also efficient for bottle washing. If you have an alternate water source, such as a well, or if lead or naturally high fluoride levels in the water are a concern, check with your baby's care team or the public health department for its recommendations.

Stroller

A stroller is valuable for carrying your baby and all your baby supplies. If your baby requires special medical equipment, purchase the best-manufactured stroller you can afford. Compare brands, and talk to other parents of babies with special needs before deciding. Look for safety features, sturdiness, storage space, and ease in collapsing and setting up. Umbrella strollers and most baby backpacks and carriers do not provide adequate support for young babies.

Nursery Audio and Video Monitors

Current nursery audio and video monitors include Wi-Fi–enabled microphones and video cameras that use a software application to connect to your smartphone or tablet and allow you to check on your baby from anywhere.

Recently, consumer products have been marketed to parents that claim to monitor their baby's heart rate and oxygen level during sleep and report the findings to a smartphone app.

At this time, the accuracy of these consumer-grade devices has not been evaluated by the US Food and Drug Administration (FDA) and they are not recommended by the American Academy of Pediatrics. If a cardiorespiratory monitor or pulse oximeter is recommended for your baby at discharge, a medical-grade device that is approved by the FDA will be prescribed by your physician.

To keep your baby safe from accidental injury—for example, strangulation by the nursery monitor cord or electrical shock from putting parts in their mouth—be sure to place the base of the monitor and other accessories out of your baby's reach, and never place this equipment near water, such as in the bathroom.

Bulletin Board, Calendar, and Journal

A bulletin board, calendar, or journal is not on most baby supply lists, but some parents of NICU graduates must keep track of a multitude of appointments and other information. Consider posting important information, such as names and contact information for your health care team, appointments, developmental milestones, medication schedules, and instructions from your physical therapist, on a bulletin board or in a journal. Figure out what will work best for you and your partner. This will become your "communication station," especially if your baby's care needs are complex. Some parents use a smartphone, notebook, or tablet, which can be taken to medical appointments, to keep track of this information as well. Having one place for all this important information will be extremely helpful when getting organized.

Arranging for Health Care After Discharge

Your baby is making good progress toward a homecoming date. You've purchased supplies and equipment, and you're comfortable with most of your baby's care tasks. Before your baby is discharged from the hospital, you need to arrange for continuing medical care.

Choosing Your Baby's Health Care Professional

Parents are sometimes caught the week before their baby's discharge without a clue as to who will provide their baby's care. If you have not yet chosen a pediatrician, begin the interviewing process well before discharge. Finding a new doctor can be an unsettling experience, especially after you've come to know and trust the hospital staff. As with any new relationship, expect a time of adjustment, uncertainty, and nervousness until trust is established. You need time to get acquainted. Your pediatrician will become an important resource person as your NICU graduate continues to grow and develop.

It is a good idea to get recommendations for a pediatrician close to home at least a couple of weeks before your baby's planned discharge. Most neonatologists do not see infants outside the NICU or intermediate care unit, but they may be able to recommend a pediatric practice in your area. Your insurance program may have a list of pediatricians. Bring the list to the hospital for help in identifying potential candidates. Nurses, close friends, or parents of NICU graduates are other possible sources of recommendations. However, if you do not have access to a pediatrician where you live, a healthy NICU graduate may be cared for by a family physician or qualified pediatric nurse practitioner. After you have a few names in hand, call and schedule a "meet the doctor" visit. Ask if this visit is free of charge or covered by your insurance because some offices will charge for this time. As you interview potential candidates, keep in mind that personality type and coping styles—yours and the doctor's—play a large part in the decision. Questions to ask are included in the " 'Meet the Doctor' Interview Questions" box.

Babies with special needs or complex health problems should have a single primary pediatrician who is able to follow their progress and coordinate their care. Choosing a pediatrician before your baby is discharged allows the physician caring for your baby in the hospital to speak directly with your pediatrician about your baby's hospital course and follow-up recommendations or send a written summary. If possible, your baby should be seen by 1 physician consistently rather than in a general health clinic where the medical personnel change often. Many pediatricians accept patients receiving public assistance if you are without private insurance. In some states, Medicaid will also provide transportation for you to take your baby to the doctor.

'Meet the Doctor' Interview Questions

- Where do you have hospital privileges? If our baby requires readmission to the hospital, will you be the primary doctor or will you refer to a hospitalist or a specialist?
- Is this your primary office location? Do you have other "satellite" offices near my home?
- What are your office hours?
- Do you provide laboratory testing in the same building, or do we need to drive to another location?
- How would I schedule an appointment?
- Who is available to answer baby care questions during the day? After hours?
- How far in advance do I need to schedule an appointment?
- How is billing handled?
- Do you care for other babies with conditions similar to my baby's? What is your training and experience with a baby like mine?
- Will other clinicians in your practice see my baby? May I meet them today?
- What procedure do we follow if we need you on a weekend or at night?
- How do we handle emergencies—should we call you first or go directly to the emergency department?
- Do you offer parent education classes?

Establishing a Medical Home

A *medical home* is a concept of care that means families and health care professionals work together as trusting partners to coordinate all of a child's care. It means having a home base for health care focused on the whole child, not just one part. In a medical home, you are valued as the expert in your child's care and treated as an important member of your child's health care team.

Your baby may go home with ongoing special health care needs. You may need help locating resources, getting referrals, making appointments, and coordinating your baby's care with several health care professionals. The doctor in your baby's medical home will be your guide during this process, helping to identify, access, and coordinate all of the medical and nonmedical services your baby needs.

Understanding Referrals

Certain specialists may continue to follow your baby after discharge. The neonatologist may call the specialist to discuss your baby's hospital course and arrange for a copy of the discharge summary to be sent to the specialist's office. Some specialists may prefer to see your baby in the hospital before discharge. The consulting physicians will usually meet with you or talk with you on the phone. They will indicate when and where follow-up examinations should occur. It is very important to attend these follow-up appointments as scheduled.

You should ask for a copy of your baby's discharge summary. Keeping a copy of this summary is helpful in case you change doctors or need to see other specialists. If your baby has complex medical problems, keep 1 in your diaper bag, or know how to access it quickly from your electronic patient portal, so you have the information handy in case of an emergency. If you have questions about anything in the summary, ask your baby's doctor or nurse practitioner.

Preparing Yourself, Your Home, and Your Family

As your baby grows and matures, you will have a lot to do. It can be overwhelming at times. Go slowly, but don't procrastinate. Preparation gives you a chance to mobilize some of your nervous energy to make a difference in your child's future.

Preparing for an Emergency

Graduates of NICUs have a higher rate of rehospitalization than the average newborn population. Common reasons for unexpected readmission are dehydration because of vomiting or diarrhea, upper respiratory infections, or hernia complications. Know which hospital you will use, if necessary, and how to get there.

If you know your baby will come home with special medical equipment, contact public services to make sure you will receive priority help during community emergencies. The emergency medical services system (or nearest fire station) and your utility providers (water, electric, and gas) should all be aware that you have a baby with special needs in your home. Ask your baby's care team about the best way to notify these services. Also be sure to notify them when your child is no longer technology dependent or if you move.

Housecleaning

Many parents feel they must do a major cleaning to eliminate germs and dust before their baby's homecoming. This is often not necessary, and families with children and pets cannot keep up an impossible level of cleanliness.

Rely on common sense as you prepare—and maintain—your home. A thorough cleaning is enough. Harsh cleaning solutions and insecticidal sprays can leave residual odors that may irritate your baby.

Tobacco Smoke

Babies—especially those who have had or are having breathing difficulties—are at risk for multiple problems from tobacco smoke. No one should smoke in the home, around your baby, or any place where your baby spends time, such as in the car. Exposure to smoke can further damage your baby's lungs, cause ear infections and hearing problems, cause hospital admission due to bronchitis or pneumonia, and increase your baby's risk for sudden infant death syndrome (SIDS).

Pets

Pets (dogs and cats in particular) can be prepared for your baby's arrival. Bring home clothing or a blanket with your baby's scent on it before your baby is discharged. Be alert for signs of aggression or jealousy when your baby comes home, and never leave your dog or cat unsupervised near your new baby. Extra attention and discipline will solve most problems.

Thinking About Child Care

If you intend to use child care within 2 or 3 months of your baby's discharge, this is a good time to start your search. The early months at home will fly by. You'll be absorbed in your baby and your family's adjustment to this new addition. While your baby is still in the hospital, you may have more time to explore the possibilities.

Babies who will need complex care require special consideration. Quality child care for infants with special needs is often hard to find, and you may face long waiting lists. For parents who plan to return to work quickly (parental leave may be used up during the NICU stay), the search for child care should begin as early as possible.

As **Ellie's** discharge approaches, Emma gets acquainted with her little sister.

Siblings

Prepare your older children for what life may be like when their baby brother or sister comes home. Plan to spend special time alone with each of your other children for a short time every day. Encourage and allow them to talk about their feelings. Most parenting books include information on helping siblings adjust to a new baby.

> "We've made a lot of progress in the past few weeks. Eden is coming home! Holland won't be far behind. Both have their feeding tubes out. Holland is a wireless baby—no more tubes or monitors! Eden will come home on oxygen and a monitor. So Holland may be the breather in the family, but Eden is the eater. Today, she took 50 mL while breastfeeding in 20 minutes."

*Billie, mother of **Holland** and **Eden***

Emotional Readiness

The days and hours before you leave the hospital are very busy and can be as stressful as the first few when you arrived. Just as you trusted the hospital staff to care for your baby, you will need to trust that they know when you and the baby are ready to go home. The staff will ensure you have the skills needed and support in place and that your baby is medically ready to transition to the next phase of life—with you as competent and loving parents.

When your baby comes home, you may experience times of great stress, nights when you'll be tempted to return your baby to the hospital, and moments when you'll wonder what you ever saw in your partner. Know that these feelings will pass. Before your baby comes home, think about things you can do to help deal with your stress. Here are a few suggestions.

▸ Exercise; talk to a counselor, religious leader, or friend; openly express your emotions (laugh and cry); or keep a journal—but do not lock in your feelings. If you are increasingly ill, accident prone, overtired, or depressed, try something different or get help.

▸ You deserve an occasional break, and couples need time alone together. Have at least 1 support person trained to babysit all of your children. If you have home nurses, take an hour or so for yourself occasionally. Have an "at-home date" while someone else is responsible for the baby's care. Do not wait for surprise breaks in the chaos or you will be too exhausted to enjoy them.

▸ Pay attention to how you manage your own anxiety about your baby and your baby's needs. It is easy to get used to being in crisis. A constant high level of worrying and watching your baby's every move is a method of trying to worry less, but it often backfires. This behavior is a sure course to burnout. Watch for changes in your baby's behavior, and develop methods of getting feedback (from a pediatrician, nurses, and friends) to help you figure things out with no panic. All in all, try to be optimistic.

▸ Be proud of your parenting abilities. Pat yourself on the back for getting this far. You have learned a lot about parenting and will continue to learn to trust your instincts as a parent.

▸ Make a list of things others could help you do. Asking for help is sometimes difficult, but this is certainly the time to do so. When people ask, "Is there anything I can do?" share your list with them. Suggestions include providing meals (freezable), shopping or running errands, doing laundry, cleaning your house, doing things with your other children, walking the dog, and doing yard work so you can rest (or play).

Rooming-in

For various reasons, you may find the prospect of taking your baby home frightening. To lessen your fear, some hospitals offer *rooming-in,* an arrangement that allows parents to stay overnight at the hospital to care for their baby independently. Nursery staff are immediately available if needed during this time. Rooming-in lets parents experience for themselves what some aspects of baby care will be like at home. Many parents feel that rooming-in builds their confidence and eases the transition to home.

Timing of the rooming-in experience is important. Ideally, rooming-in should take place as close to discharge as possible. To simulate the home environment, try to have any home monitoring equipment in place during rooming-in. Rooming-in for parents who must learn about special medical equipment might be necessary for several days.

You may wish to complete your rooming-in experience a day or two before your baby's discharge date. A good night's sleep the night before discharge may help ease some of the inevitable anxiety of your baby's homecoming.

Celebrating

Last but not least, celebrate your baby's upcoming arrival home. When your baby's health care team finally sets a discharge date, consider planning a celebration dinner with your partner before your baby is discharged. Once your baby comes home, it may be a few weeks or more before you can find much quality "couple time" in your schedules.

Isaac and **Eliza** pose for a photo in their going-home outfits. (They did not share a crib in the hospital.)

Discharge Day at Last!

Discharge day is exciting and frightening at the same time. Even the most prepared parents feel nervous about finally bringing their baby home.

Be prepared for delays on discharge day. You may arrive first thing in the morning, only to be told you'll have to wait for 1 more test, for the results of a previous test, or for a member of your baby's care team to examine your baby or write an order.

> " There was so much anticipation and buildup for our son's discharge from the NICU that by the time the day arrived, I was surprised by my sudden sadness to leave the place I so desperately wanted to flee. "
>
> *Robyn, mother of **Auggie***

When everything is finally in place, ask for a written or an electronic copy of the baby's discharge summary. Some NICUs send a copy to your pediatrician. Dress your baby in the special going-home clothes you've brought with you, and ask if you may take a brief tour through the unit so the team can say good-bye and celebrate with you.

Some parents want to do something special for the staff. Thank-you cards, a letter to the hospital administrator expressing appreciation for the NICU and nursery staff, and letters and photos from home are the most valuable gifts you can give the staff. They enjoy seeing the progress your baby makes.

Now you're on your way out the door with discharge instructions and bags of supplies, toys, and baby clothes. Don't forget your baby!

Alex left the NICU after 126 days.

Niklas, Gabbie, & Lukas

Born at 28 weeks, 4 days

In late 2006, at 28 weeks 4 days' gestation, our weekly ultrasound ended abruptly and we were escorted to a "comfy" room with flowery wallpaper to wait for the doctor. It turned out that triplet C was being deprived of the proper nutrients to survive, forcing us to make a choice to either continue with the pregnancy, knowing that triplet C would die within the next 48 hours, or have an emergency C-section. We chose the latter. Lukas was born weighing 1 pound 12 ounces, and Gabbie and Niklas were just over 2 pounds.

While waiting with Greta in the recovery room, I was told I could go visit the babies. As I was gazing at my daughter lying in the incubator, I commented to one of the nurses about the cute little baby noises she was making. I was gently told that those noises I was hearing were grunts. She was struggling to breathe and it turned out her lung had collapsed. In the course of a couple days, all 3 moved to oscillating ventilators that mechanically moved their chests up and down. Within a few hours after birth, our babies had developed life-threatening respiratory distress syndrome, collapsed lungs, patent ductus arteriosus, and jaundice, and each kid suffered at least one pneumothorax (collapsed lung). Niklas developed pulmonary interstitial emphysema, and we were told it would be appropriate to say good-bye to him. He was so sick that we never actually put his crib together, as we didn't want to go through the pain of taking it apart upon his death.

About 1 week in, we received the worst news. Niklas had developed 2 brain bleeds, one in each hemisphere of his brain (an intraventricular hemorrhage)—a grade III on one side and a grade IV on the other. Grades I and II are most common, and often there are no further complications. Grades III and IV are the most serious and usually result in long-term brain injury to the infant. After a grade III or IV hemorrhage, blood clots may form, which can block the flow of cerebrospinal fluid, leading to increased fluid in the brain (hydrocephalus).

The triplets in the NICU. (The practice of co-bedding is not observed anymore.)

The doctors watched carefully, hoping that this situation would resolve itself. It did not. A temporary shunt was installed while we continued to see if it would resolve. It did not. A permanent shunt was then installed, which required 3 more brain surgeries to get correct. After the last surgery, we were told to expect poor eyesight, possible blindness, and likely cerebral palsy and learning disabilities. Niklas had sunset eyes after the surgery, where the irises made him look as though he was staring down—an unsettling look that we were told was permanent. After 3 months in the NICU, we brought the kids home, along with their oxygen tanks.

Today, the sunset eyes and the oxygen tanks are gone. The physical and cognitive impairments that were once certainties never transpired. In fact, not one of our 3 kids even wears glasses. We feel very blessed that our babies were in the skilled hands of the doctors and nurses in the NICU.

Today, they are 9 years old, and we are very busy with school and after-school activities. For the most part, the triplets are average busy third graders who attend a Catholic school and enjoy learning Spanish after school. All 3 test average or above average at school.

In winter, all 3 are alpine ski enthusiasts and belong to the ski team. When ski season is over, we swim and water-ski. Last year, both boys attended sailing camp and have become good little sailors with hopes to attend the same camp again for many summers. Niklas loves taking classes and has shown an unusual talent in guitar as well as tae kwon do. Lukas is quite good at swimming and tae kwon do. Gabbie has been taking ballet classes since she was 4 years old and enjoys them to this day. Also, all 3 enjoy playing tennis.

To our pleasant surprise, all 3 have been really healthy. They don't even get common colds. I am a true believer in encouraging outdoor activities in the fresh air, sticking to strict sleep schedules, and eating a very clean diet of local or organic foods. **Read more about Niklas, Gabbie, and Lukas in "Where Are They Now?" in the Appendix.**

Jason and Greta, parents of Niklas, Gabbie, & Lukas

The triplets, at age 9.

CHAPTER 9

Home at Last

> **"** I was honestly excited but also very scared about bringing Abel home after 7 months. I was so scared of the fact that I was taking him from the only home he had ever known and people who were with him daily when I was not, and afraid that we were not going to have a strong bond. But I quickly found out that I am capable of taking care of my son. Our connection is very strong and it has grown since being able to spend more quality time with him.
>
> *Shana, mother of **Abel***

Welcome home! Your phone is ringing, your baby is crying, your children are screaming, your dog is barking, your dishes and laundry are piling up—it all seems to be too much to handle.

Bringing your baby (or babies) home can be overwhelming. All of the other demands of everyday life will be waiting for you, along with your new baby and their special care needs.

While your baby was in the hospital, your primary focus was on learning about the NICU, the new medical language and routines, and how to meet your baby's immediate needs. If you were able to spend a lot of time learning to care for your baby in the NICU, you have probably become quite good at the basics. If you were not able to be with your baby often, you probably received a lot of instructions before your baby was discharged. In either instance, you may find that once you get home, everything turns into chaos. Relax! This is normal for anyone with a new baby in the house, even for experienced parents. It's especially true for parents of preterm babies or others with special needs.

Parenting any baby, especially one born at risk, demands an enormous amount of adjustment. Most parents can't wait for their baby (or babies) to come home, but even the most experienced and prepared parents find the first few weeks a huge challenge.

Homecoming: You, Your Children, and Your Visitors

Even though you're relieved your baby is home, you may find that you miss the support of the hospital staff. You may feel alone and abandoned as you make the adjustment to independent parenting. For some parents, the first days at home with the baby are as stressful as their first days in the NICU.

Anxiety

You may feel highly anxious now that you have total responsibility for your baby's care and feel as though you don't remember a single thing you were taught about caring for your baby.

It may be comforting to know that you now share something with parents of healthy newborns: feelings of uncertainty and clumsiness regarding baby care at home. Your anxiety should diminish as you find that you are, indeed, surviving. You may do things differently than they were done in the hospital, but as long as the decisions you make keep your baby safe and thriving, you can have confidence in them.

> After 100 days in the NICU, the doctors gave us the okay to go home. We should have been excited but instead, we were hesitant and nervous since Eliana would be coming home on oxygen and a feeding tube. There were so many what-ifs, but the nurses and doctors reassured us and gave us confidence that we were ready and able to take care of our baby. Being at home turned out to feel so normal.

*Sophany and Mike, parents of **Eliana***

Grief and Guilt

When you first started your NICU journey, you were probably told that your baby's problems were not your fault and were, in fact, outside anyone's control. Yet you may have felt guilty anyway and said to yourself, "If only I had …" Soon, though, your busy life as a NICU parent overshadowed these feelings.

Now that your baby is home, feelings of sadness and guilt may return. Parents may feel guilty when they grieve for what might have been instead of feeling grateful for the baby they have.

These feelings of grief and guilt usually pass as you gain confidence caring for your baby and adjust to your role as a parent. Support from your family, friends, and health care professionals is important to getting through this stage. Keep in mind that your own mental health goes hand in hand with your baby's healthy growth and development. Talk to someone familiar with your NICU experience; this may help with your feelings of loss of the healthy term baby you had expected.

If these feelings persist or if you continue to have upsetting memories of the NICU experience, seek help from a health care professional.

> " I wish someone would have talked to me about what mental health challenges I might expect in the days, weeks, and months after we left the NICU. Posttraumatic stress, whether it reaches the level of disorder or not, is common among NICU parents. That trauma for me didn't really kick in until after we went home. He'd gone into respiratory failure in my arms, so it's not surprising that I started having panic attacks. I worried, What if these treatments worked, but only for a short time? When we got home, I would look at him and think, Well, now he's dead. I had these thoughts many times each day and night. I was able to find a therapist who specialized in early parenthood transitions. She and the other members of my medical team were invaluable to turning my experience around and moving forward. "
>
> *Alex, father of* **Pascal**

Love and Attachment

The bonds you established with your baby during hospitalization are very real. But development of true intimacy may have been difficult because of the lack of privacy and the distrac-

tions of hospital technology. Now that you are at home, your baby may suddenly seem like a little stranger. You may worry if you do not have strong feelings of love toward your baby.

Give yourself some time to get to know your baby—and to let your baby get to know you. At first, your baby will make incredible demands on your time and attention and seem to give back little. But as your baby grows, you will notice that your baby responds to your efforts with quiet alertness, more frequent eye contact, and that first amazing smile. All relationships take time to grow, and with time your love for your baby will grow.

After leaving the hospital, **Logan** and his mother appreciate quiet time at home.

Feeling Overwhelmed

It is not realistic to think that only 1 or 2 people can parent a baby 24 hours a day, 7 days a week. Make a plan ahead of time so you can call on trusted friends and family to help you by caring for your baby on very stressful days when you need a breather.

There is nothing bad about feeling as though you are going to "lose it" with your baby. The important thing is to recognize when you have reached your limit. Put your baby in a safe place, such as the crib, and close the door. Take a deep breath and put your support plan into action.

Call a person who has agreed to help you and listen to you when you need to talk. If you do not have this kind of support, call your pediatrician's office, a parent support hotline, or call or text 988 to reach the Suicide & Crisis Lifeline. They can help you make a plan for keeping your baby safe while you take a few minutes to calm down.

> ❝ Holland liked to cuddle, but at first, she fussed a bit more, and it took more trial and error to figure out what she wanted. Both girls were pretty good-natured, but I must admit that I am **not** supermom! There were nights when I was so tired and cranky that my babies and I just sat and cried together! ❞
>
> *Billie, mother of **Holland** and **Eden***

Effect on Your Older Children

The reality of the baby's homecoming is stressful for most siblings. Once the baby is home, your other children may be surprised that your attention is still focused so intensely on the baby. You can help children adjust to their new role as older brothers and sisters by suggesting activities such as a special dinner or dessert just to celebrate this new status as an older sibling. If you can, give a small gift to each older sibling the day you bring your NICU graduate home. Involve your children's teachers, too—perhaps by sending a photo of the baby for the big brother or sister to show to classmates in a special moment.

As your children watch the baby take even more of your time, attention, and love, you may notice they seem angry at you or the baby, regress to thumb-sucking or bed-wetting, act out to get your attention, or have difficulty at school.

If older children are interested, involve them in the care of the new baby as much as possible, even though this may sometimes mean more work for you. Try not to criticize any "help" you receive, and praise a job well done. The more you can include older children in caregiving, the sooner they will adjust to the new baby's presence.

Spend some special time alone with each child, even if just for a few minutes of snuggling, reading a book, playing a game, or taking a walk together. The addition of a new baby changes your relationship with your other children, and working through this adjustment together is an important part of your growth as a parent and family.

Visitors

When your baby comes home, your friends and neighbors may assume the crisis is over and be less available for support. On the other hand, friends who were nowhere to be found during your NICU crisis may now knock on your door to see your new baby and expect to be treated as visitors.

Most health care professionals and parents of NICU graduates will tell you to limit visitors. The more people your baby is exposed to, the greater the risk of infection. Healthy visitors may be welcome, but anyone with a fever, cold, cough, open sore (such as a fever blister), or other contagious illness should not be allowed near the baby. No one should touch your baby or your baby's belongings without first washing their hands. Good handwashing is the best protection against illness. Most people understand when you explain that a common illness picked up from an older child or adult can develop into a serious infection for a NICU graduate.

You probably won't want to discourage all visitors because you'll need help now that your baby is home. Now more than ever, you may need to make a list of things people can do to help you, such as running errands, helping with laundry, or watching your children while you nap. Now is not the time to be super parent—ask for and accept help!

What to Expect From Your Baby

Babies are unique in the way they react to their surroundings and signal their needs. A large part of gaining confidence as a parent is feeling you are adequately meeting your baby's needs. Parenting a NICU graduate can be challenging at first, especially if your baby does not signal those needs clearly or does not act predictably.

Preterm Babies Are Different

Compared with term babies of a similar age, preterm babies are sometimes more irritable, less responsive, and less predictable. Term babies with chronic illnesses requiring NICU time may behave this way too.

Try to be patient. Most babies outgrow these differences within the first year after birth and grow into typical toddlers. Until that time, however, your baby may try your patience. By understanding your baby's behavior and helping your baby become more organized, you'll find it easier to get into a routine.

An important part of caring for your baby is learning what is normal and understanding how to recognize a change. A parent is often the first and best person to recognize a change in the baby's general condition, including positive changes and potential concerns or changes in behavior, which should be brought to the doctor's attention.

Corrected Age

If your baby was born early, there are 2 important days to mark on the calendar. The day your baby was born is the official date of birth, but your baby's estimated due date is also an important day. When you measure your baby's development—that is, when you look at what is "normal" for your baby's age—consider both of these dates. By looking at the difference between them, you can adjust your baby's calendar age to account for prematurity and calculate your baby's *corrected age*. During the first 2 years, using the corrected age will give you a better idea when your baby should reach common developmental goals.

Calculating corrected age isn't difficult. Begin with your baby's actual age in weeks (number of weeks since the date of birth) and then subtract the number of weeks your baby was preterm. This is your baby's corrected age. A term pregnancy is 40 weeks' gestation. To determine the number of weeks preterm at birth, subtract the baby's gestational age in weeks at birth from 40. For example, if your baby was born at 32 weeks' gestation, your baby was 8 weeks preterm. If your baby is now 16 weeks old, the corrected age is 8 weeks. As your baby gets older, it may be easier to make the correction in months (4 weeks = 1 month).

Actual age in weeks minus	Weeks preterm	=	Corrected age
16 weeks since birth –	8 weeks	=	8 weeks

In this case, even if your preterm baby is 16 weeks old, you should expect your baby to have developmental skills similar to those of 8-week-old term babies, like starting to smile and holding their head up. It would be unrealistic to expect your baby to be ready to roll over from the stomach to the back, a skill that often develops in term babies around the age of 16 weeks.

Parents are often frustrated by well-meaning family and friends who express concerns about their baby's development. People may think your baby is delayed for a 4-month-old, for example, when, in fact, your baby is perfectly on target for a baby with a corrected age of 2 months.

Sleep Patterns

Don't expect your preterm baby to sleep through the night for many months. Unlike a term baby, who might sleep a full 6 to 8 hours at night by 4 months of age, your baby may not sleep through the night until 6 to 8 months of age or later. Until a regular sleep cycle develops, help

your baby to fall asleep at night by separating daytime and nighttime activities. Talk and play with your baby during daytime awake periods. Keep night feedings calm and quiet. This will help your baby learn the difference between day and night and may help you get much-needed sleep. Try to put your baby to bed on their back when your baby is drowsy but still awake. Becoming used to falling asleep without someone in the room may help your baby fall back to sleep if awoken during the night. How the baby is positioned for sleep is very important. Lying the baby flat on their back without additional blankets, pillows, stuffed animals, or crib bumpers reduces the risk of sudden infant death syndrome (SIDS). For more information on SIDS, see the Sudden Infant Death (SIDS) section later in this chapter.

Babies vary in how easily they settle down to sleep. Follow the same steps each time you put your baby down to sleep to help the baby learn a personal going-to-sleep routine.

"We were lucky. Auggie was always smiling and so happy."

Robyn, mother of **Auggie**

> ❝ Abel is a wonderful baby and sleeps through the night. My husband and I do not. Abel gets his first medication at 5 am. His feedings begin at 6 am and continue for 90 minutes every 3 hours until midnight. We do our best sleeping between 2 am and 5 am. ❞
>
> *Shana, mother of **Abel***

Fussing and Crying

Although your baby will sleep up to 16 hours a day at first, the actual sleep times may be short. Your baby may awaken and fuss every 2 to 3 hours until 3 to 4 months' corrected age even if not hungry.

Try holding your baby with the baby's arms and legs tucked closely to the body and rocking the baby while you stand or sit in a rocking chair. Some babies prefer a gentle up-and-down motion instead of side-to-side movement. Your baby may prefer a walk in your arms or in a stroller or carriage. Some babies find a rocking swing comforting, but only use a swing if your baby passed the car safety seat test, has no respiratory problems in a sitting position, and is big enough to sit safely. Other babies like singing and hearing music or "white noise" from a vacuum cleaner, clothes dryer, or fan. A warm bath may be calming. Still others enjoy being gently patted, massaged, held skin-to-skin on your chest, swaddled snugly (but not too tightly), or going for a ride in the car. Many babies find sucking on their hand or a pacifier comforting. Try one thing at a time and you'll learn what works best.

If your baby is unusually fussy or will not settle down, check to see if something could be causing pain (for example, the sharp edge of a clothing tag, a hair wrapped tightly around a finger or toe, an eyelash in your baby's eye) and check for fever or other signs of illness.

Many babies go through a fussy or colicky period that begins anywhere from 2 to 4 weeks' corrected age, peaks around 6 weeks' corrected age, and often resolves by 3 months' corrected age but can last until 6 months' corrected age. For some babies, this fussy period occurs at the same time every day (usually late afternoon or early evening). Fussy periods also happen when your baby is eating while becoming more alert and aware of the environment. In other words, your baby becomes overwhelmed by the end of the day and needs a good cry to relax! But getting your baby to calm down may be a challenge.

During your baby's first months at home, you'll be learning what things your baby likes and doesn't like. The most frustrating thing for parents is that the same comfort measure doesn't work every time—and may not work 2 times in a row. When you find something that works, stick with it until it doesn't work any longer. Babies often like consistency and rituals, especially as they get older.

How long to let your baby cry remains controversial. If your baby has special needs and turns blue with crying, your choice is clear and you need to respond quickly. If your baby is healthy, you can make a parenting choice. Some experts believe that babies should never be allowed to cry it out alone. They advise parents to respond quickly to their babies to meet their need for security and to let them know they are important. Some babies seem to need to cry themselves to sleep and will not be comforted no matter what you try.

This controversial aspect of baby care can be an important topic to discuss with your pediatrician. Whether you decide to respond to your baby's cry immediately or wait a moment, the important thing is to do what you feel is right. You can try a combination of approaches before deciding which one is right for you and your baby. If your baby is very fussy every day, make a plan for someone to give you a break, even if only for an hour or so. You will need a break so you can return to your baby feeling more relaxed and calm.

Concerns About Feeding

Now that your baby is home, you'll be making more independent decisions about when and how much your baby eats. Some parents discover things they didn't learn about their baby's eating habits while the baby was in the hospital and wonder if they are "doing it right" at home.

Breastfeeding your preterm baby or baby with special needs at home can be challenging. You can use the resources available in your community, including your pediatrician, a lactation consultant, or a support group, to help you stay inspired and confident in your abilities.

Helping Your Baby Eat Well

A calm place to eat is important for all babies but especially for those who become stressed from too much stimulation. Watch your baby's cues during the feeding. Does your baby yawn, sneeze, hiccup, get frantic, or lose interest and fall asleep in the middle of feeding? Talking into your baby's face or feeding your baby near the television may be too much for your baby to handle.

Lucy shows how much she's grown by posing next to her preemie outfit.

> ❝ Lucy could not breastfeed when she was discharged and it took her another 2 months after we came home to get it. At 17 months old, it is definitely her favorite pastime. This is so hard to believe after what a struggle it once was for her. ❞
>
> *Kate, mother of **Lucy***

Tips for a Successful Feeding Experience

- If you are feeding your baby formula, prepare the formula in advance.

- If you warm the formula or breast milk, do not use a microwave oven because the bottle may be heated unevenly and you could scald your baby's mouth. Place the bottle in hot water or a bottle warmer instead, and check the temperature of the milk against your wrist to make sure it is lukewarm.

- Minimize distractions in the room. Dim the lights a bit and turn down the television or radio.

- Support your baby's head, neck, and hips, flexing the hips slightly.

- To help your baby anticipate the feeding, place your finger or a few drops of breast milk or formula on the baby's lips.

- If necessary, gently support your baby's jaw with your finger to keep the milk in the baby's mouth.

- Find the right bottle and nipple for your baby. You should know this before hospital discharge.

- Watch for signs of stress, and give your baby a break when necessary.

- Give your baby quiet time to recover after the feeding is over.

- Never put your baby to sleep with a bottle propped in the baby's mouth or allow your baby to sleep with a bottle. Your baby could easily choke, and bottle propping leads to baby tooth decay and, possibly, ear infections.

How Much and How Often to Feed

Before your baby's discharge, the NICU team should have explained the feeding plan and provided you with written instructions. These instructions probably included how much and how often to feed your baby. Special preterm discharge formulas designed specifically for growing preterm babies are sometimes continued after discharge to help with weight gain during the transition to home. Some babies need a specific feeding schedule after discharge. Your pediatrician may adjust that schedule only after weighing and examining your baby in the office. Other babies may be able to feed *on demand* or *ad lib,* meaning the baby determines how much and how often to eat.

"Instead of a nasogastric tube, Abel has a G-tube in his abdomen because he aspirates easily. He gets his G-tube feeding every 3 hours, takes 5 to 10 mL of breast milk in a bottle several times a day for practice, and then he can practice breastfeeding after I pump."

*Shana, mother of **Abel***

If you will be feeding your baby on demand at home, you should begin to feed this way before discharge. This will give you an opportunity to learn your baby's cues that signal readiness to eat. If your baby's feeding cues are not fully mature at the time of discharge, the recommendation may be to feed your baby on demand but offer a feeding at least every 3 to 4 hours, with a minimum of 6 to 8 feedings per day.

Your NICU team may suggest a combination of feeding methods for your growing baby at the time of discharge. You may be asked to breastfeed for a certain number of feedings each day, use an alternate method for the other feedings, and gradually increase the frequency of breastfeeding while your baby's weight gain is monitored. Between breastfeeding sessions, you can provide either breast milk or formula by using a bottle or supplemental nursing device, finger feeding, or cup feeding. Whenever you are supplementing your baby's feedings (with breast milk or formula), it is important for the breastfeeding parent to continue to pump milk after every feeding to maintain or build the milk supply. Supplementation without pumping allows your baby to be fed but does not provide the stimulation necessary to continue making milk.

As your baby grows, so should their appetite. If your baby takes less than what's needed at a feeding, they may wake up earlier or take more at the next feeding. Once your baby is able to take in more at each feeding, the time between feedings may lengthen. It's particularly nice when your baby starts lengthening the time between feedings at night, letting you get more sleep.

Feeding schedules need to be individualized based on your baby's feeding ability and weight gain. Visits with your pediatrician, home health nurse, or a lactation specialist during the first week or two after discharge (and for as long as necessary after that) can help resolve any ongoing feeding issues.

How Long to Feed

Feeding length varies, depending on how frequently your baby wants to eat and how easily your baby tires while feeding. Breastfed babies may begin nursing only a few minutes on each side and may require more frequent feedings. You should hear sucking and swallowing, along with some pauses. Gradually, your baby may work up to nursing 20 minutes or more on each side. The usual length of time needed to complete a feeding is about 20 minutes. Healthy preterm newborns who do not have any health issues, especially respiratory problems, may want to nurse for up to 40 minutes. As long as your baby does not seem exhausted, seems content after feeding, and is gaining weight (weight checks may need to be done at home or in the doctor's office), there's no reason to limit feeding time. In fact, your baby may become frustrated if you end the feeding too soon. Babies nurse not only to satisfy hunger but also to satisfy their need for sucking, security, and comfort. Falling asleep or ceasing to suck are the usual indicators that a feeding is over.

In general, a feeding by bottle finishes more quickly than a feeding at the breast, but this also depends on how vigorously the baby sucks and swallows and how often the baby needs to take a break. Some NICU graduates feed from the bottle until they become tired (you will recognize these signs from learning to feed your baby in the NICU) and finish the feeding with a feeding tube. Your baby will gain strength gradually and you'll notice improved feeding abilities, so there is no need to push your baby. Your baby will have more difficulty gaining weight if burning calories to get through long, perhaps stressful, feeding sessions.

Weight Gain

As you settle into a feeding routine, you may wonder whether your baby is gaining enough weight. Optimal weight gain is approximately 15 g (½ oz) per day before your baby's due date and 20 to 30 g (a little more than ½ to 1 oz) per day for the next 6 months. You're aiming for a weight gain of 1 lb per month. Your baby's pediatrician will plot weight, length, and head circumference measurements on a growth chart and may recommend weekly weight checks at the office or at home by a visiting nurse for the first few weeks (or longer) after discharge.

Feeding Problems

Some babies are more difficult to feed than others. Even though you practiced feeding your baby in the hospital, some problems may persist after your baby comes home.

A bottle-feeding baby who gulps rapidly and then spits everything up may need a nipple that delivers the milk more slowly. You might need to try a few different types of standard bottle nipples before you find the one that works best. You may need to regulate the length of time the nipple is in your baby's mouth as well. Frequent burping and feeding the baby in a more upright position may also help prevent spitting up.

If your baby tends to gulp food or stop breathing during feedings, your NICU nurse probably helped you watch the breathing patterns and your baby's color during feedings. Preterm babies frequently have trouble coordinating sucking, swallowing, and breathing during a feeding. If you notice breath holding or a color change (to pale, dusky, or blue) at any time during a feeding, take the nipple out of your baby's mouth. Try gentle stimulation—rubbing or patting your baby's back, for example—to remind your baby to breathe. The rubbing or patting may also bring up a burp. As preterm babies mature, their coordination improves. If this is a new behavior for your baby or your baby is having more frequent breathing difficulty during feedings, call your pediatrician at once.

If you have difficulty feeding your baby after discharge, contact your pediatrician. Frequently, all you need is some advice and reassurance from a health care professional who is familiar with your baby's eating habits.

A Feeding Log

Whether your baby is breastfeeding or bottle-feeding, you may want to keep a log of each feeding for the first few weeks at home. Keeping a log is a simple and valuable way to work in partnership with your baby's pediatrician. Use a notebook to document

- Feeding times
- Time at breast or amount per bottle
- Any feeding difficulties
- Wet and dirty diapers
- Special comments (for example, is your baby satisfied after a feeding or does your baby cry a lot; does your baby fall asleep in the middle of the feeding; does your baby need to be awakened for feedings?)

Bring this information with you when you take your baby to the pediatrician. Appointments at the pediatrician's office are often only 15 minutes long, giving you little time to organize your questions. If you come prepared with your written questions and feeding log, you will be able to make the most of your office visit. Once your baby has established a consistent pattern of feeding and gaining weight at home, you can comfortably retire your feeding log as part of your baby book.

Other Common Homecoming Concerns

It may have seemed like an eternity until you were able to take your baby home. Now, at last, you have control over your baby and your family life—or do you? The normal elements of baby care may not be so routine for you. The first few days, weeks, and even months at home may, in fact, be unsettling. Here are some common concerns, with the goal of helping you to organize your family life once again.

> **Try your hardest to not look back. Look forward with your baby (or babies!). Forgive yourself if you're carrying guilt and focus on taking care of yourself, your baby, and your partner now.**
>
> *Kate, mother of **Lucy***

Sudden Infant Death Syndrome (SIDS)

Many parents worry about their baby's chances of dying from SIDS, sometimes called *crib death*. *Sudden infant death syndrome* is the sudden death of a baby younger than 1 year that doesn't

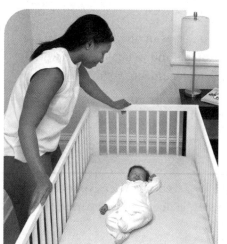

have a known cause even after a complete investigation. While in a sleep environment, babies can also die from accidental causes, such as accidental suffocation or strangulation, or from ill-defined causes.

Your baby should sleep on their back on a firm mattress covered with a fitted sheet. There should be no other bedding or soft objects in the sleep area.

*Image courtesy of the Safe to Sleep® campaign, for educational purposes only; Eunice Kennedy Shriver National Institute of Child Health and Human Development, **http://safetosleep.nichd.nih.gov**; Safe to Sleep® is a registered trademark of the US Department of Health and Human Services.*

Reducing the Risk of SIDS and Sleep-Related Deaths

There are several things you can do to create a safe sleep environment for your baby.

▸ Always place your baby to sleep on their back, for naps and at night.

▸ Place your baby in a safety-approved crib or bassinet, on a firm mattress, with a properly fitted sheet. There should be no other bedding or soft objects in the sleep area.

▸ Your baby should not sleep in an adult bed, on a couch, or on a chair alone, with you, or with anyone else.

▸ Blankets should not be used for "nesting" or to provide boundaries for your baby.

▸ If your baby falls asleep in a car safety seat, a stroller, a swing, or an infant carrier, the baby should be moved to a firm sleep surface as soon as possible.

▸ Avoid sleep positioning devices sold to parents with the claim that they position babies for safe sleep or that are inconsistent with safe sleep recommendations.

▸ Keep all blankets, sheepskins, cushions, quilts, comforters, fluffy or loose bedding, beanbags, and stuffed toys out of your baby's crib.

▸ Make sure nothing is covering your baby's head.

▸ Share a room with your baby for the first 6 months. Give your baby their own sleep space (crib, bassinet, or portable play yard) in your room, separate from your bed. Share your room, but don't share your bed.

▸ Breastfeed your baby.

▸ Offer a dry pacifier at sleep time throughout the first year after birth. If your baby doesn't want it or if it falls out of their mouth, do not force it or prop the pacifier in place. Do not hang the pacifier around your baby's neck, and do not attach the pacifier to your baby's clothing while sleeping.

▸ Don't smoke or let anyone else smoke or vape around your baby. If you smoke, talk with your doctor about getting help to quit.

▸ Don't overdress or over-bundle your baby and don't overheat your baby's room. Your baby should be lightly clothed or in a sleep sack, and the bedroom temperature should feel comfortable to a lightly clothed adult. Your baby should not feel hot to the touch and should not be sweating.

▸ Home cardiorespiratory monitors do not reduce the risk of SIDS.

All babies, including preterm and low-birth-weight babies, should be placed on their back to sleep. You may have seen babies lying on their stomach in the NICU surrounded by rolled blankets. This was done at an earlier time in the baby's life for specific medical reasons when the baby was on continuous heart rate and respiratory monitoring. This should not be done at home. A small number of babies with special medical conditions may sleep in a different position, but your baby's pediatrician will discuss this with you.

For additional information about how to decrease the risk of SIDS and sleep-related deaths, visit the official American Academy of Pediatrics (AAP) website for parents: **www.HealthyChildren.org/safesleep**.

Please use this QR code to go directly to www.HealthyChildren.org/safesleep.

Concerns About Back Sleeping

Most new parents are aware of the recommendations for positioning babies on their back to sleep. Your parents or grandparents, however, raised "tummy sleepers" and may have the following concerns about back sleeping:

- **Choking:** The most common fear about the back-sleeping position is that the baby will spit up and choke while asleep. Healthy NICU graduates can turn their heads or protect their airways if they spit up, so choking while sleeping on their back should not be a concern.
- **Flat head:** Technically called *positional plagiocephaly,* preterm babies' heads are often flat in the back and narrow on the sides. As they mature, hold their head up independently, and spend less time on their back, their head usually rounds out. Encourage plenty of supervised tummy time when your baby is awake, and avoid placing your baby in car safety seat carriers or "bouncers" for long lengths of time. Frequently change the shoulder you use to hold your baby, the position your baby faces in the crib, and the direction the crib faces in the room so your baby is not always turned onto the same side. If plagiocephaly occurs despite these preventive measures, talk with your pediatrician about possible treatment options.
- **Delayed development:** Allowing your baby plenty of supervised tummy time while awake will build the necessary neck and shoulder muscles needed to roll over.

Family Bed: Not Recommended

Your friends may have shared their bed with their newborn or young children. As research emerged on *SIDS* risk factors, the American Academy of Pediatrics determined that the safest place for your baby to sleep is in the room where you sleep but not in your bed and not in the same bed as another baby.

Placing your baby's crib or bassinet near your bed (within arm's reach) will make breastfeeding easier and allow you to better watch over your baby. This is especially true for parents of babies who require frequent nighttime feedings or who have special needs, such as medical treatments around the clock. Sudden infant death syndrome prevention studies recommend that babies should sleep in their parents' room for the first 6 months.

Alex (left) builds muscle during tummy time so that he can lift his chest off the floor with his arms. **Eliana** (right) takes a little break after working hard during her tummy time.

"Our lives now are busy, busy, busy, and without much sleep. The babies never sleep for more than a 3-hour stretch. It was OK at first, but that kind of sleeping schedule really catches up with you. When they wake up at 4:00 am, it takes over an hour for us to warm bottles, feed and burp, pump, and clean up, so I don't get back to sleep until around 5:15 am, only to wake up again around 7:45 am. I guess that's the life of a mommy. On top of all that normal baby stuff, we are also dealing with 2 to 3 doctor appointments a week, medicine schedules, and all kinds of equipment and alarms."

*Billie, mother of **Holland** and **Eden***

Bathing

As long as your baby's face, neck, skinfolds, and diaper area are clean, you don't have to bathe your baby every day. A sponge bath will be fine until your baby can tolerate a tub bath without much stress. Some parents get into the tub with their baby to hold and snuggle as they wash. This provides skin-to-skin contact for you and your baby. Hold your baby securely and be sure the bathwater isn't too hot for your baby.

There are only 2 rules for tub bathing your baby: Don't let your baby get cold, and keep your baby safe.

Never leave your baby unattended in the tub. If the doorbell rings and you must answer it, wrap your baby in a towel and bring your baby with you. If you must reach for something or turn away, keep one hand securely on your baby.

Bathe your baby in the warmest area of the house—preferably one free from drafts. You'll need only a few inches of water that feels comfortably warm to your wrist or elbow. Your baby will be slippery when wet; try placing a soft towel or preformed sponge insert in the bottom of the tub. Use a mild soap to wash your baby's body. No soap is needed on your baby's face. Most pediatricians advise against the routine use of lotions and powders.

If your son was circumcised, you were probably instructed not to tub bathe him until the circumcision is healed. If you chose not to have your baby circumcised, you simply need to wash the penis at bath time. Don't try to pull back the foreskin. It will naturally separate from the penis over several years, and as your son grows, you'll teach him to wash carefully as part of his daily routine.

> ❝ We are learning that there will never be a solid routine. Every day is different. Maybe the meds change or he pushes a faster feed cycle or is having a rough day and we need to add more time and adjust everything else accordingly. So I would say that after your baby comes home, act just as you did during the hospital stay: Take it day by day and just care for your child the best way you can. ❞
>
> *Shana, mother of **Abel***

Keeping Your Baby Warm Enough

Before discharge, you learned how to take your baby's temperature. Unless you've been instructed to check your baby's temperature routinely, you'll probably take it only when you suspect illness. But how can you tell if your baby is maintaining a comfortable body temperature?

It's not necessary (and not recommended) to turn your heat up to an uncomfortable level to keep your baby warm. A normal household temperature that is comfortable for an adult in light clothing is recommended for most babies. If you have special concerns, ask your baby's pediatrician for advice.

Dress your baby in the same clothing or one more layer than you would wear to feel comfortable. If you're comfortable in a T-shirt and shorts, for example, your baby may need a footed jumper suit. On a cooler day, when you need a shirt and a pullover sweater, dress your baby in a jumper suit and a sweater. Avoid the temptation to overdress (and overheat) your baby. A baby who is dressed too warmly may fuss, turn red, and possibly sweat. The temperature of a baby's hands or feet may not be reliable, but if the baby's tummy feels cool, add a layer of clothing.

Outings

Use common sense when deciding about outings. There's probably no reason why your baby can't sit outside in the shade with you on a nice spring day or go with you to a healthy friend's house for lunch. Avoid any exposure to direct sunlight in the spring and summer months. Even a short period in direct sun can result in sunburn at this stage.

Most health care professionals suggest limiting your baby's exposures for the first 1 to 2 months at home. Fall and winter months are especially bad for cold and flu viruses that could put your NICU graduate back into the hospital, but contagious viruses are even present in the spring and summer months. If you do take your baby out, avoid crowded places and limit the number of people who have direct contact with your baby. Anyone who touches your baby must first wash their hands or use an alcohol-based hand sanitizer.

Lucy is secured safely in her car seat for one of her first outings.

> 66 I learned a lot from the nurses—to change and then feed instead of the other way around, the amazingness of swaddling, the miracle of diaper rash cream. Even Pascal's struggle with the car seat test taught me a lot about car seat safety and getting a baby positioned well. I wouldn't be the dad I am without the NICU. 99
>
> *Alex, father of* **Pascal**

Babysitters and Child Care

Because you may limit your baby's outings and visitors for the first few months at home, you may be wondering what to do when you need to go out. Anyone who watches your baby while you are away, whether that person is a babysitter, grandparent, or other relative or friend, should know how to manage your baby's needs and understand safe sleep positioning. Ideally, all of your babysitters should complete an infant cardiopulmonary resuscitation (CPR) course. Some hospitals offer CPR courses for NICU parents and caregivers. If your hospital does not offer a CPR course, consider using the American Heart Association/AAP *Infant CPR Anytime* program. This is a self-directed personal training kit that allows anyone to learn how to perform infant CPR in about 20 minutes.

Check your babysitter's references and ask about previous child care experience. If you are using out-of-home child care, it is important to look carefully at the child care facilities in your area and consider some important points.

Choosing Child Care for Your Baby

- Choose a state-certified/licensed child care facility and make sure that every child care worker is certified in infant and child CPR according to American Heart Association guidelines.

- Check with consumer groups and your state's licensing authority to make sure there have been no unresolved complaints or health violations made against the facility.

- Ask the director about infant sleep position practices and if the facility has ever cared for infants who were born preterm or have special needs.

- Ask about visitation policies. You should be allowed to visit the facility anytime so you can really see staff interact with infants and toddlers. Some facilities have special webcams so you can view your baby at any time during the day while you are at work.

- Pay particular attention to child care workers' handwashing practices and whether they use gloves when changing diapers. Are there sinks and soap near the cribs?

- Look at the storage area for breast milk and formula. Are bottles clearly labeled? What precautions are taken to decrease the risk of feeding a baby the wrong formula or someone else's breast milk?

- What is the caregiver-to-baby ratio? The lower the ratio, the better it is for your preterm baby or NICU graduate. Keep in mind that child care centers that foster developmental care and offer low worker-to-baby ratios tend to be more expensive and in demand and have longer waiting lists.

- For more information on choosing a quality child care center, visit the official AAP website for parents: **www.HealthyChildren.org**.

Secondhand and Thirdhand Smoke

Secondhand smoke is exhaled smoke and the smoke that comes from the tip of a burning cigarette, pipe, or cigar. It contains thousands of dangerous chemicals, with more than 50 of them known to cause cancer. Thirdhand smoke is the contamination that remains after the cigarette is put out. Thirdhand smoke is found on the clothing and furniture of a smoker and in the car where a smoker uses tobacco. Anytime your baby is near someone who has been smoking, your baby is exposed to these chemicals (as are you).

Babies and children exposed to smoke from these sources have a higher risk of developing serious health problems, including *SIDS,* ear infections, respiratory problems, allergies, and asthma.

It is important to create a smoke-free environment for you, your baby, and your family. Ban smoking in your house (put a sign on your front door as a reminder if necessary) and anyplace where your baby spends time. If your baby's caregivers smoke, they should change their clothes or cover their clothing after smoking and before they come near your baby. Avoid places that are not smoke-free and be aware that secondhand and thirdhand smoke is damaging to your baby's health and development.

Protecting Your Baby From Illness

Many parents feel like paramedics in training throughout their children's lives. The first fever, the first rash, the first fall off the tricycle all present new experiences in assessment and treatment. The possibility of illness is especially frightening for parents of preterm babies or babies with special needs, who have already had to overcome many obstacles just to get home. Most parents learn, through experience, the difference between serious and minor problems.

Strategies to Avoid Illness

Good handwashing is the single best way to prevent the spread of infection. Always wash your hands (and your other children's hands) when you arrive home from work, child care, or school. Wash your hands after you change a diaper and, of course, after you use the bathroom.

You know to limit visitors soon after your baby's arrival home and to ask friends or family with illnesses not to visit. But what if you or someone in your household gets sick? How do you keep your baby from getting the illness?

If possible, someone who is not sick should do most of the baby care if you are sick. Keeping ill siblings away from their baby sister or brother can be difficult; it may be easier to keep the baby away from them. A careful explanation may help if the ill child is old enough to understand that your baby could easily catch the illness.

> Holland was in the hospital with pneumonia, and then sick again with a cold and an ear infection a mere 3 weeks later! We went back on lockdown! No one visited unless they had been symptom free for at least 48 hours, and anyone who approached our babies had to wash their hands! It's one thing when you have a normal kid who gets a cold and gets over it. It's a whole different scene when you have to worry that your kid is going to end up in the hospital because she can't breathe with every little cold she gets.

*Billie, mother of **Holland** and **Eden***

Good handwashing is particularly important if you or someone in your family has a cold, the flu, a fever, or a stomach or diarrheal illness. Wash your hands before you pick up your baby and before breastfeeding or preparing a bottle. Covering coughs and sneezes and keeping hands clean can help prevent the spread of serious respiratory illnesses. To help stop the spread of germs, cover your mouth and nose with a tissue when you cough or sneeze, throw used tissues in the trash, and cough or sneeze into your elbow instead of your hands if you don't have a tissue. Remember to immediately wash your hands after blowing your nose, coughing, or sneezing. Do not allow sick people to kiss or get too close to the baby's face, especially if they have a respiratory infection or cold sore (fever blister). If a person with a respiratory infection must be near your baby, consider having them wear a mask.

Keep everyone in your family and those who have frequent contact with your baby up to date on their immunizations. This is an easy step to protect your baby from preventable, and often devastating, diseases (see Chapter 8).

Working With Your Baby's Pediatrician

If your baby is a healthy NICU graduate with few or no complications, most illnesses will run their course without problems. If your baby was very preterm or has ongoing health problems at home, illness may represent a greater threat.

Ask your pediatrician when you should call about a suspected illness. If your baby has special health needs, discuss the kind of problems that can be expected and which ones can be managed at home. Seeing your pediatrician on a regular basis for the first few months gives you the opportunity to obtain answers to all of your what-if questions and may avoid anxious visits to the emergency department in the middle of the night.

Knowing how much care and monitoring your baby required in the NICU, you may be concerned you won't be able to tell when your baby is getting sick at home. All babies get sick, but not every illness is life-threatening. You'll quickly learn your baby's normal behavior and will be the best person to determine when something is not right. Trust your instincts.

Signs of Illness to Report to Your Pediatrician

Some signs of illness include

- Fever (a temperature higher than 100.4°F [38°C] rectally). The rectal route is recommended until your baby reaches at least 6 months of age (or until your pediatrician gives you the go-ahead to use a different route).

- Difficulty breathing (faster and harder, using more effort or grunting, noisy breathing)

- Lack of interest in eating or not feeding as well as usual

- Vomiting most or all feedings (different from the usual amount if your baby frequently spits up food) or vomit that is green or bloody

- Watery stools that soak into the diaper

- More crying and irritability than usual (calming and comforting don't work as usual) or refusal to sleep

- Change in color: pale, bluish, or blotchy (*mottled*) appearance

- Behavior that is "just not right"; for example, less activity than usual, more sleeping, more difficulty waking

---

It's important to know when your baby is not acting normally, but you aren't expected to be the doctor. When you have concerns about illness, call your pediatrician. Most offices expect calls from concerned parents and have experienced staff ready to help you. If you call after hours and get the answering service, be sure to include any special circumstances with your baby (for example, say that your baby is a NICU graduate on home oxygen) in case a pediatrician who is not familiar with your baby's history receives the message. That will help ensure a speedy response to your call.

Be ready to supply the following information:

▶ Why you think your baby is ill

▶ The baby's temperature and how you took the temperature (A rectal temperature is most accurate in a baby.)

▶ Current medications, any new medications or recently discontinued medications, and recent immunizations

Taking Your Baby's Temperature

In the NICU, your baby's temperature was taken many times a day, and usually under your baby's arm. If this screening measurement was unusually high or low, the nurse verified the measurement by taking a rectal temperature, which is the most accurate method for determining your baby's temperature.

Taking a rectal temperature

After your baby is home, if you suspect your baby has a fever, your pediatrician will probably ask you to take a rectal temperature.

Place your baby's tummy over your legs or on a firm surface, such as a changing table. This lets you control your baby's movements and prevents your baby from rolling onto the thermometer, which could cause an injury.

1/2"

The thermometer should be inserted one-half inch into the rectum. Never force a rectal thermometer.

Ask your pediatrician which type of thermometer is recommended for your NICU graduate.

Giving Medications: Missed or Vomited Doses

If your baby must take medications at home, you need to know the name, purpose, dose (how much), when, how, and for how long to give each medication to your baby. You should know any special instructions, like whether the medicine should be taken with food, and possible side effects or reactions. You should know if there are any special instructions for storing the medicine. You should have received this information before discharge. Tack this information to your bulletin board or tape it to your refrigerator door for handy reference and keep a copy with you.

Give all medications as directed by your baby's doctor. Most medications work best when a steady level is maintained in the body. If you forget a dose of medicine and it is only a couple of hours late, give it as soon as possible and count it as "on time." However, if it is more than halfway to the next time a dose is due (for example, a dose is given every 12 hours and you are more than 6 hours late, or a dose is given every 6 hours and you are more than 3 hours late), skip the missed dose and get back to your regular schedule with the next dose. If you have any questions, check with your baby's doctor or nurse. Never try to make up for a missed dose by doubling or increasing the next dose.

If your baby vomits within 30 minutes after you give a dose, repeat the full dose. If your baby vomits more than 30 minutes after you give a dose, do not give a repeat dose. It is difficult to know how much of the drug was absorbed and you do not want to give a double dose. Missing one dose of a medication is usually not a problem. If you have any questions, check with your baby's doctor or nurse. Never try to make up for a vomited dose by doubling or increasing the next dose.

Call your doctor if your baby misses or vomits 2 regularly scheduled doses or if your baby begins to vomit more feedings than usual. Also notify your doctor if your baby experiences any of the potential adverse effects associated with a medication.

Basic Rules for Medications

Don't forget these basic rules about medications.

- Keep all medications out of the reach of children.
- Use the dosing device (syringe or medicine cup) that came with the medicine. Do not use your regular silverware or household measuring spoons to estimate a dose.
- Do not give your baby nonprescription medicines without asking your baby's doctor, especially cough and cold syrups, which may have side effects that are dangerous to your baby.
- Fever medicine, such as acetaminophen (for example, Tylenol) or ibuprofen (for example, Advil), should not be given to babies younger than 3 months without first asking a health care professional. Never give your baby aspirin.
- Do not use old prescription medicines or another child's prescription medicine.
- Find out how to store the medication; for example, some medicines require refrigeration.
- Always use child-resistant safety caps.
- Talk to your pediatrician if you have any questions.
- Do not give medication in the dark. Be sure you have enough light to read the label, measure the dose, and see that your baby actually took the medication.
- If you think your child has taken the wrong medicine or too much of a medicine, call poison control at 800/222-1222.

On Your Own

Your baby's homecoming is a big event. Homecoming is also an adjustment—a time of shifting values, expectations, and priorities. Parents of NICU graduates have all the concerns of parents of healthy term babies, and then some. Don't isolate yourself and try to handle everything alone. Find people who can and will support you. Take a moment to appreciate those who have helped you get to this point, and be proud of all you have learned about caring for your new baby.

Allison

&

Reece

Born at 33 weeks

Born just shy of 33 weeks, Allison and Reece were 3 pounds 7 ounces and 4 pounds 8 ounces, respectively. Allison's water broke at 28 weeks, but with close monitoring, doctors were able to help delay their births for 5 weeks. While this was a very scary and uncertain time for us and their siblings, it was priceless for their development. An infection eventually called for an emergency C-section. They spent almost a month in the NICU, first receiving respiratory care and treatment for jaundice, and then focusing on growing and learning to eat. The circumstances resulted in a disappointing breastfeeding experience. We also faced the challenges of different NICU release dates, but in the end, the result of 2 healthy, happy children is priceless!

Reece and Allison, at 15 days old.

From the beginning, Allison and Reece have been distinctly different individuals. Allison, with big, expressive eyes, always needed more attention as a baby, while Reece was more easygoing and a better sleeper. As they became toddlers, Allison was the alpha twin who showed more independence and mothered Reece, while Reece was happy to follow along. He also had some speech delays but is on track now. While they fight, as all siblings do, they play well together using their amazing imaginations, and their twin bond is unquestionable.

Allison creates elaborate scenes with her dolls and ponies, while Reece prefers things with wheels and learning facts about "our world." Together, they craft endlessly and love to be outside. **Read more about Allison and Reece in "Where Are They Now?" in the Appendix.**

Gudrun, mother of Allison & Reece

Reece and Allison.

Jack

Born at 29 weeks

&

Henry

Born at 31 weeks

Jack

- Born in 2009
- Weight: 2 pounds 11 ounces
- Length: 15 inches
- Gestational age: 29 weeks
- NICU stay: 56 days

Jack had a number of complications when he was born, mainly breathing issues. He was on and off a ventilator for the first few days. He did go home on oxygen and a monitor. He also had monthly follow-ups with the developmental clinic to monitor his progress.

Today, Jack is a happy, healthy 6-year-old. He has had no long-term complications or issues due to his early start to life. Jack was in speech therapy for 2 years, but any issues have since resolved. He is an active kindergartner who loves to play with Legos, draw, and ice-skate. Jack has a fondness for music and has even started taking guitar lessons. When we tell people that Jack was a preemie, most are surprised because of how well he is doing. We've come a long way from the long days in the NICU and will forever be grateful to the medical team that helped Jack and us.

Jack was born at 29 weeks' gestation in 2009.

Henry

- Born in 2012, 2 years and 3 months after his brother Jack
- Weight: 3 pounds 7 ounces
- Gestational age: 31 weeks
- NICU stay: 47 days

Henry was born with issues common for a baby at his gestation, mainly breathing. He was on continuous positive airway pressure (CPAP) for a short time and was able to wean to a nasal cannula after a few days. Henry's course in the NICU was uneventful when compared to our other son, Jack, which we were grateful for. He went home without oxygen and no specialist follow-up. Today, Henry is a rambunctious 3½-year-old. He is definitely our "active" child who loves to run and play sports. He started soccer last fall and will continue this spring. His favorite sports are soccer, baseball, and ice-skating. He has no long-term complications or issues due to his early start. He is currently in speech therapy but has progressed quickly and will be stopping soon. As with Jack, we are amazed and forever grateful to the wonderful medical team and staff during Henry's stay in the NICU. **Read more about Jack and Henry in "Where Are They Now?" in the Appendix.**

Kristina, mother of Jack & Henry

Henry was born at 31 weeks' gestation.

Jack, at age 6 years, and his brother, Henry, at age 3½ years.

As Your Child Grows

> " Having a baby in the NICU was probably one of the hardest things we've ever had to go through, but truly worth all the tears, all the driving back and forth, all the back pains from sleeping on the hospital couch, all the meals we had to eat at the hospital, and all the questions we had to ask many times over because we didn't understand. We made lasting friendships, we have our miracle baby, and we have an incredible story to tell.
>
> *Sophany and Mike, parents of **Eliana*** "

The NICU experience doesn't end when you arrive home. Many parents describe their child's first year after birth as the longest roller-coaster ride of their lives. The first weeks at home are filled with mixed emotions, new challenges, and changes within your family. Now that you're home and settled into a routine, you'll begin looking to the future.

"Will My Child Be Normal?"

Having a baby in the NICU can be a frightening experience, and your initial concerns may have focused on whether your baby would survive. Once your child is medically stable, though, it's only natural to wonder, "Will my child be normal?" Knowing what kind of follow-up to expect for your child and how you can contribute to your child's progress are rewarding aspects of parenting a NICU graduate.

You play an extremely important role in your child's growth and development. Loving interactions with attentive parents can help children who were born preterm or with other health problems achieve optimum development. This chapter addresses how parents can monitor their children's development and things they can do to help them reach their full potential.

Risk Factors

Many parents worry about their child's risk of ongoing health problems, possible physical challenges, and learning delays. Studies show that NICU graduates have a higher risk of health issues and learning or developmental delays during infancy and early childhood compared with babies who do not need NICU care. Usually, the lower a newborn's birth weight and the more complicated the hospital stay, the greater the risk of future problems.

Some of the factors that put babies at higher risk are a birth weight less than 1,500 g (3 lb 5 oz)—also called very low birth weight—brain injury (bleeding in the brain or damage to the developing nervous system), poor head growth, chronic lung disease (bronchopulmonary dysplasia), serious vision loss, certain genetic syndromes, and abnormal muscle tone (limp or stiff muscles).

Take advantage of the moments when your baby is alert to talk to them, sing songs, and socialize.

Parenting and the Learning Environment

Of course, medical problems are not the only factors determining a child's developmental outcome. Environment plays an important role in health and learning. Supportive parenting, stimulation, and an environment rich in learning opportunities are important for children's growth and development.

This does not mean you have to buy expensive toys that claim to make infants and toddlers smarter. Your child needs to be loved and nurtured. Infants and toddlers can learn a lot from the people around them and from an environment that's naturally rich with learning opportunities for a curious mind. Parents who share simple activities with their children, like talking, singing, reading a book, and imitating each other's facial expressions, provide important stimulation and opportunities to learn.

Developmental Milestones and Your Child

Developmental milestones are the skills or achievements that your child develops in predictable steps over time. For example, typical milestones that you will watch for include social skills, like making eye contact and smiling; large muscle (motor) skills, like babies bringing their hands to their mouth; and small muscle skills, like grasping objects. Typically, babies develop large muscle skills from the head down. For example, babies usually develop head control before they learn to roll over, sit, or crawl. Although developmental milestones follow patterns that you can monitor, children develop at their own speed and in their own way.

Watching for Progress

It is a good idea to keep your own record of your child's progress. When trying to spot a delay in developing milestones, it is helpful to know the signs of typical development. Many books describe infant development and have places to keep track of developmental milestones. The American Academy of Pediatrics official website for parents has an online AAP Motor Delay Tool (**www.healthychildren.org/English/MotorDelay/Pages/default.aspx**) that includes an interactive checklist of milestones that educates parents about physical development in babies and young children. It can serve as a guide if you have a feeling that something is wrong, and you can print out a checklist of items to start a conversation with your pediatrician.

Please use this QR code to go directly to
www.healthychildren.org/English/MotorDelay/Pages/default.aspx.

Other reliable sources of information include the Centers for Disease Control and Prevention (**www.cdc.gov/milestones**), which provides checklists to help you track your child's progress. Whether you use a book or an online checklist, bring your record to all of your follow-up medical appointments so information can be shared with your baby's pediatrician or developmental specialist.

Please use this QR code to go directly to
www.cdc.gov/milestones.

If your baby was born prematurely, remember to adjust your baby's age to get a better sense of which developmental milestones are expected. Subtract the number of weeks your baby was born early from your baby's actual age in weeks (number of weeks since birth). For example, if your baby is 24 weeks today but was born 10 weeks early, your baby's corrected age is 14 weeks (24 weeks minus 10 weeks = 14 weeks). This means you should be looking at the milestones listed under the 3- to 4-month (12–16 week) section. Use this corrected age when you look at developmental milestones for the first 2 years of your child's life. (See Chapter 9 for more information about corrected age.)

Another important factor in developmental progress is the presence of chronic illness. Even if brain development is normal, children with severe lung disease, heart disease, or intestinal problems may have delays because they cannot physically handle some activities. This may be especially apparent in skills involving large muscles.

As you watch your child's development, remember that children follow similar patterns but do not always learn the same things at the same times. Children develop skills at their own pace and may reach milestones in different ways. Even healthy term infants achieve developmental milestones over a range of ages. Some children are walking by 9 months and others, not until 15 months. This will be especially true for preterm babies. Some babies are more assertive, more active, and quicker to learn, and, therefore, may develop at a faster pace than babies who are content to observe and quietly socialize. Your child may not meet each of the developmental milestones at the time described on the checklist. The most important thing is ensuring that your child continues to make progress and achieve new milestones.

"I feel sad at moments like these, when my smooshy little babies seem too grown up. I feel sad because I didn't take enough time to enjoy them. Their babyhood was so full of overwhelming stress, anxiety, sadness, and worry that it was hard to keep my head above water. Looking back, I wish I had been able to spend less time worrying over every silly milestone and had just enjoyed the little snickerdoodles that they were."

Billie, mother of **Holland** *and* **Eden**

Optimizing Your Baby's Early Development

Understanding Your Baby

Every baby is different and might achieve developmental milestones in different ways. Take time to think about your baby and answer the questions in the box titled "Understanding Your Baby's Early Development." Your answers will help you understand your baby and how your baby is growing.

Understanding Your Baby's Early Development

- How does my baby let me know what they are thinking and feeling?

- How does my baby let me know when they have had enough and need a nap?

- Is my baby naturally louder and more active or naturally quieter and less active?

- How does my baby like to explore the world? Does my baby prefer to use fingers and hands (small muscles) or arms and legs (big muscles)?

- What kinds of objects and activities interest my baby?

- How does my baby respond to new situations? Does my baby prefer to look around before feeling safe, or jump right in? Does my baby need frequent breaks from lots of sights and sounds, or does my baby stay calm?

- What are my baby's strengths?

- In what ways does my baby need more support?

Adapted from American Academy of Pediatrics. *Supporting You and Your Preemie: Milestone Guidelines for Premature Babies.* American Academy of Pediatrics; 2008.

Things You Can Do

You are your baby's most important teacher. As your baby grows, you will have many opportunities to teach different skills. Over time, parents learn to couple realistic expectations of their baby's abilities with support and inspiration for their baby to stretch their skills and reach their potential. Suggestions for fostering your baby's development are included in the box titled "Ways to Optimize Your Baby's Early Development." If many of these suggestions seem like simple common sense, you are already on the right track to optimizing your baby's development!

> " I'm constantly advocating for services that Abel needs for his growth and development, and that our family needs for mental health and financial stability. Our social worker continues to be very helpful with these issues. "

Shana, mother of **Abel**

Ways to Optimize Your Baby's Early Development

- Talk, smile, make happy sounds, laugh, and socialize with your baby.
- Sing songs to your baby.
- Read books to your baby.
- Respond to your baby's smile or babbling with your own smile, touch, or voice.
- Change your baby's position during play, including sitting and lying on the back or stomach.
- Offer toys and other objects that your baby must reach for.
- Bring your baby's hands together to the center of their body and allow your baby to bring their hands to their mouth.
- When your baby can hold objects, encourage your baby to make sounds by banging objects together.
- When your baby is approaching 6 months' corrected age, place your baby on their back and place toys out of their reach on 1 side to encourage rolling onto the stomach.
- When your baby is approaching 9 months' corrected age, play social games (patty-cake) and name objects in sight to encourage vocabulary development.
- Praise and encourage your baby's efforts.

Shana optimizes **Abel's** development by making happy sounds, laughing, and socializing during play time.

Developmental Follow-up

At the time of discharge from the NICU, you and your baby may be referred to a developmental follow-up clinic at the same hospital or a different one in the region. You may also be given a referral to your community's early intervention program. Your pediatrician will be monitoring your baby's development and making any necessary referrals.

In the developmental follow-up clinic, you may see several specialists with knowledge about different aspects of growth and development. The specialists will look at how your baby moves, plays, and interacts with them. Like the list you use at home, the specialists use a variety of screening tests to score your baby's activity.

When **Auggie** goes to a restaurant with his parents, he has the opportunity to learn about his environment and to expand his vocabulary and social skills.

"When Kellan was 2 years old, our doctor told us that, on average, 2-year-olds should have a vocabulary of around 50 words. Kellan had about 10 words. We were shocked. Our pediatrician assured us that even though Kellan had not been accepted into the early intervention program a year ago, we should call and have him evaluated again. The speech therapist came to our house, and after the evaluation, we were excited to hear her say, 'I can't wait to work with Kellan.' She came to our house once a month for a year and Kellan went from 10 words to speaking in full sentences in no time. This picture was taken shortly after Kellan turned 3 and graduated from his therapy and headed off to preschool."

*Marnie, mother of **Kellan***

Individuals With Disabilities Education Act and Early Intervention

Because the foundation for learning begins in early infancy, every baby identified as at risk for developmental delay should receive intervention as early as possible. The Individuals With Disabilities Education Act (IDEA) is a law that ensures children with disabilities receive important services, including support and assistance for the family (**https://sites.ed.gov/idea**). You can find contact information for the IDEA lead in your state on the IDEA website. The Early Intervention (EI) program is a federal grant run by individual states that works with children up to age 3 years who are at risk for developmental delays.

Please use this QR code to go directly to https://sites.ed.gov/idea.

You may be eligible for services if your child experiences any difficulties with physical, mental, language, social, hearing, visual, behavioral, or emotional skills. Anyone can refer a child to the local EI program. You may have received a referral from the hospital, or your pediatrician may make a referral if any developmental concerns arise during office visits. You can even refer your child to your local EI program by going to **www.cdc.gov/findEI** or calling 800/CDC-INFO (800/232-4636) and asking how to contact your state's EI program.

Please use this QR code to go directly to www.cdc.gov/findEI.

Once a referral is made, the EI program team of specialists will gather information about your child and family to determine your needs. If the team determines that your child needs services, an Individualized Family Service Program (IFSP) will be developed. The IFSP explains the services that are recommended for your child and how the EI program will help. Depending on your child's needs, services such as occupational therapy, physical therapy, speech therapy, social work, or nursing care may be provided in your home or at a center. Your IFSP should be reviewed by you and your service coordinator at least every 6 months and modified as your child's needs change. You may request a review earlier if you feel your child needs more services or has outgrown the need for therapy. If therapies are still needed at 3 years of age, your child will transition from EI and an IFSP to an Individualized Education Program and preschool services through your local school system.

Payment for EI services varies from state to state, but all states must provide at least some services free of charge. You can obtain information about your state EI program from your pediatrician, your state's department of health, your local health district, or the Early Childhood Technical Assistance Center website (**http://ectacenter.org**).

Please use this QR code to go directly to http://ectacenter.org.

Therapy professionals can teach you developmentally appropriate ways to play with your child, and they may teach you special exercises to strengthen your child's muscles or positioning techniques if your child has any physical disabilities. Enjoy working with your child and take pride in knowing you are making an important difference in your child's development.

"Logan has grown into a very tall, very active 5-year-old who loves drawing, nature, and animals. He is currently deciding if he will be a geologist or botanist when he grows up. He is one of my favorite people and I could not imagine life without him."

*Christina, mother of **Logan***

Problems That May Worry You

As children get older, some may face ongoing developmental or physical challenges. Although many NICU graduates have no long-term health or developmental problems, it is important to know the types of problems that some NICU graduates have so you can watch for them and intervene early. Work with your child's pediatrician, therapists, and teachers to identify any areas of concern and find the right resources for help. You are not alone.

Learning Problems

Some NICU graduates experience learning problems, including problems with drawing and writing, language development, following directions, and reading comprehension. Children who experience these problems in school may require special education classes to assist their learning. Almost half of very-low-birth-weight babies receive some form of special education in school. The percentage of babies diagnosed with an intellectual disability increases as gestational age and birth weight decrease. At school age, very preterm babies are at a 2- to 5-times higher risk of having an intellectual disability compared with a healthy full-term baby, but the type of disability ranges widely from very mild to severe. Attempting to predict whether a baby will have an intellectual disability at school age is difficult when the baby is very young. A variety of developmental testing tools are available to evaluate older infants and toddlers.

Cerebral Palsy

Cerebral palsy (CP) is a diagnosis that many parents of preterm babies fear. It is an abnormality of muscle movement or tone caused by a malformation or damage to the nerve cells in the brain. Babies with CP have muscles that are too stiff or too limp and have poor coordination. The frequency of CP is higher in the smallest and most preterm babies and occurs in approximately 1 in 10 babies born weighing less than 1,500 g (3 lb 5 oz).

Cerebral palsy does not mean there is a problem with intelligence, although some children with CP also have learning disabilities. The diagnosis of CP is generally not made until the preterm infant is 12 to 18 months' corrected age unless the infant's problems are severe. In some infants, muscle tone is increased (called *spasticity* or *hypertonia*); in others, muscles are abnormally limp (*hypotonia*). *Spastic diplegia,* or stiff muscle tone of the legs and arms, with more involvement of legs and feet, is the most common form of CP among preterm infants. Many preterm infants with this type of CP have normal to near-normal intelligence. *Spastic quadriplegia* is when all 4 extremities, along with the head and trunk, are fairly equally affected. This is the most severe form of CP and often can be diagnosed before the first year after birth. Spastic quadriplegia is frequently associated with intellectual disability. Thus, the characteristics of CP can range from mild muscle tone abnormalities with normal or above-average intelligence to severe physical and intellectual disability.

Signs of CP can vary because of the different types and degree of disability. Some of the early clues your child may have CP focus on delays in achieving motor milestones. Some of the early warning signs are in the box titled "Warning Signs of Cerebral Palsy." When looking at your child for these signs, be sure to use your child's age corrected for prematurity.

Warning Signs of Cerebral Palsy

Younger than 6 months
- When cradled in your arms, your baby always seems to push away from you, overextending their back and neck.
- When you pick your baby up, their legs get stiff, and cross each other or "scissor."

6 to 10 months old
- Your baby reaches out with only 1 hand while keeping the other hand fisted.

Older than 10 months
- Your baby is lopsided when crawling, pushing off with only 1 hand and leg while dragging the opposite hand and leg.
- Your baby scoots around on their buttocks but does not crawl on all fours.

Adapted from American Academy of Pediatrics. *Caring for Your Baby and Young Child: Birth to Age 5*. 5th ed. Shelov SP, Altmann TR, eds. Bantam Books; 2009.

Children diagnosed with CP need close developmental follow-up and referrals to an EI program. In addition to a developmental pediatrician, children with CP may be referred to pediatric neurology (brain), orthopedic (bone and joint), and physical medicine/rehabilitation specialists to plan their treatment.

Alex at age 19 months

Alex at 3½ years old

"**Alex** has gone through intensive physical and occupational therapy since discharge. He eats anything and everything by mouth. He continues to see several specialists for cerebral palsy and spastic diplegia. He is walking with an irregular gait, but he is fully walking, climbing, running, and keeping up with his 2 brothers and his friends."

*Stacy, mother of **Alex***

> I've been thinking, pondering, wondering. How do I teach Eden that she is just like everyone else? That her disability does not define her? That she can do whatever she wants, based on her strengths? That everyone has strengths and weaknesses?
>
> How do I teach others that she is a 'normal' kid? That she should be treated the same as everyone else? That she loves all the same things that the other kids like? That she wants to play too?
>
> Then it hit me ... she is **not** like everyone else.
>
> If I fail to recognize and accept her differences, if I fail to recognize and embrace her many strengths, I am failing her. She is different. Just like everyone else.

*Billie, mother of **Holland** and **Eden***

Vision and Hearing Problems

Graduates from the NICU, especially the tiniest and most preterm babies, are at risk for future vision and hearing problems.

Children with severe retinopathy of prematurity (ROP) have the highest risk of serious vision problems. Even though most children with ROP get better over time and never need treatment, a small number of children born preterm lose their vision from ROP. Continued follow-up with your child's eye doctor until the ROP is resolved is extremely important to prevent serious visual loss or blindness.

Children born very preterm also have an increased risk of nearsightedness and crossed or lazy eyes. The risk is highest in children who previously had severe ROP or significant bleeding in their brain. Because vision is so important for achieving developmental milestones, children with visual problems need evaluation by a pediatric eye doctor (ophthalmologist), developmental follow-up, and EI, Early Intervention program.

Graduates from the NICU also have a higher risk of hearing loss. Even though studies show hearing loss is much more common in children born preterm than in those born full term, the chance is quite small. Between 1 and 4 of every 100 children born very preterm will have

serious hearing loss requiring a hearing aid. Hearing problems can also occur in children who had persistent pulmonary hypertension of the newborn, hypoxic-ischemic encephalopathy, severe jaundice (hyperbilirubinemia), or infections or who received medications that can affect the ear (certain antibiotics and diuretics). All NICU graduates have their hearing screened before hospital discharge, but hearing loss may not be discovered until later. If you have any concerns that your child is not hearing normally, talk with your pediatrician.

"Holland is awfully cute in her new pink glasses. She looks so grown-up and studious. We could tell when she first put them on that she knew something was different."

*Billie, mother of **Holland** and **Eden***

Behavior Problems

Not all preterm or chronically ill babies have behavior problems in childhood, but some do. Children who were born preterm or have been chronically ill may be less able to handle stimulation and exhibit unpredictable feeding, crying, and sleeping patterns. Behavior problems seen in early childhood include frequent temper tantrums, overaggressiveness in play, hyperactivity, and exaggerated separation anxiety. Children may be extra sensitive to loud sounds or certain textures that are touched or eaten. Parents may need to learn their special behavioral cues to prevent overstimulation.

As children reach school age, their behaviors may worsen or they may improve with maturity. Some children have discipline problems because of a short attention span, hyperactivity, and disorganized behavior. Others may show more introverted behavior, with extreme shyness and anxiety. If your child develops behavioral problems, close follow-up and teamwork with your pediatrician and schoolteachers are important.

Allowing Your NICU Graduate to Grow Up

Graduates of the NICU may come home with nursing support, equipment, supplies, medications, and a long list of caregiving requirements. You may have been given a list of dos and don'ts for your baby's care and warned of the potential for rehospitalization. It's no wonder that at first, you tend to overprotect your baby. In some cases, though, this sheltering continues well past the point of necessity and beyond what is healthy for you and your child.

> " During our NICU stay, I saved 1 diaper of every size to help me see how the twins were growing. Now my twins take a very small diaper for show-and-tell during Superhero Week at school. They say, 'My superpower is I was able to fit into this tiny diaper. What is your superpower?'
>
> *Parina, mother of **Isaac** and **Eliza***

Vulnerable Child Syndrome

When parents continue to view their children as sickly despite healthy findings on physical examinations, they may be experiencing something called *vulnerable child syndrome*. At

school age, they do not allow their children to participate in sports or special events. The parents don't encourage high academic standards, and so their healthy children perform below their potential.

Overprotection stunts children's efforts to develop skills appropriate for their age. They may continue to experience separation anxiety and have temper tantrums whenever they do not get their way. They may have difficulty playing with or participating in games with other children. They may bite or hit other children during outbursts of anger.

Professional intervention is often necessary to help parents recognize and accept that the illness event, which took place years earlier, is now over. Only then can these parents begin to view their children as healthy individuals and encourage their social development.

Colson is bright-eyed and eager for adventure.

A Difficult Balance

After being in the NICU, it is completely understandable that you want to protect your child. Caring for and protecting your baby without providing too much care and protection is, indeed, a tricky balancing act. You've worked hard to get to this point, and it's only natural to want to safeguard your special baby. Close watchfulness may be necessary and appropriate early in life because of continued medical problems. But part of being a parent is growing with your child and realizing when it's time to loosen your grip in some areas and expect your child's cooperation in others. Listen to your pediatrician and other child care specialists when they tell you your child is medically stable and developmentally ready for new challenges.

Exploring the world and feeling accomplished as an individual is important for all children. You'll find your own way as you give your child's abilities a chance to develop and unfold. Through trial and error, you'll learn how much to expect from your child and when the time is right to stretch those expectations a bit further. Although every child is different, most children benefit when their parents encourage accomplishments that reflect their fullest abilities.

"**Meridith** is a smart, loving, resilient, strong young lady who is thriving!"

*Mary Ellen, mother of **Meridith***

Ellie's first birthday!

Working With Your Pediatrician

Remember that you are not alone. Your pediatrician is your partner and is dedicated to helping you meet your child's health and developmental needs. If you have concerns about your child, start by talking with your pediatrician. You may be asked to complete some additional screening questionnaires. Your observations are an important part of your pediatrician's evaluation. If a specific diagnosis is found, your pediatrician can help you connect with resources or special support groups in your community.

Talking to Your Pediatrician About Your Child's Development

Helpful tips

- When making the appointment, tell the office staff that you have concerns about your child's development and want to discuss them with the doctor.

- Bring a list of your questions, concerns, and any examples you can think of.

- Fill out 1 of the milestone checklists from the American Academy of Pediatrics official website for parents (**https://www.healthychildren.org/English/MotorDelay/Pages/default.aspx**)

Please use this QR code to go directly to https://www.healthychildren.org/English/MotorDelay/Pages/default.aspx.

or from the Centers for Disease Control and Prevention (**www.cdc.gov/milestones**).

Please use this QR code to go directly to www.cdc.gov/milestones.

- Ask another adult who knows your child to fill out the milestone checklist too.

- If you can, take another adult with you to play with your child so you can focus on what your doctor says.

Ask all of your questions during the visit.

- Tell your doctor that you have concerns right at the start of the visit and share the checklist and questions that you wrote down.

- If your doctor is in a hurry that day, ask if you can schedule another visit.

- Ask your doctor about the results of the most recent developmental screening.

- Take notes to help you remember what your doctor says.

Make sure you understand the next steps.

- Before you leave, make sure your questions have been answered.

- If you don't understand something, ask your doctor to explain it again or in a different way.

- Make sure you know the next steps and have the information you need. For example, do you need to make an appointment with a specialist? Do you have the phone number? Do you need a written referral?

- Review your notes when you get home and call the doctor's office if you have more questions.

Adapted from Centers for Disease Control and Prevention. Learn the Signs. Act Early. http://www.cdc.gov/actearly. Updated September 19, 2022.

Believing in Yourself

Many parents of NICU graduates are a bit frightened to look far ahead. In fact, fear of the unknown contributes to chronic stress in many families. The potential for rehospitalization, future health problems, and overprotection of your child is very real.

The NICU experience does not make for an easy transition to parenthood. As your child grows, you'll continue to discover important parenting resources within yourself—for managing stress, advocating for your child's needs, and seeking support and lending it to those around you. For you, parenthood has brought unique changes that are different from those experienced by parents whose babies were born healthy. It's given you opportunities for building relationships, uncovering hidden strengths, and reordering priorities.

"Auggie had his first boating adventure at about 18 months. He thoroughly enjoyed it."

*Robyn, mother of **Auggie***

"Eliana is 2 years old and growing, running, climbing, talking, learning, and as feisty as ever. We've had many appointments with the neonatologists, ophthalmologists, physical and occupational therapists, and a speech therapist—all working together to get her where she needs to be."

*Sophany and Mike, parents of **Eliana***

You may face many challenges ahead. But you can feel good about your parenting if you continue to ask questions and actively participate with the health care team as your child's advocate.

What happened to your baby before birth and in the NICU is an important part of your child's medical legacy. It plays a role in your child's growth and development, but it is not the only important factor. The way parents raise their children has the potential to change the course of their future health, growth, and development. A parent's most difficult task is knowing when to offer a helping hand, and when to provide a gentle push forward. Your job is to inspire achievement and independence, while realizing that some of life's most valuable lessons come from disappointment. Trust yourself to have a positive effect on your child's life. The NICU experience created unique challenges for you and your child. Take a moment to reflect on what you've achieved and congratulate yourself for a job well done.

The next chapter discusses the loss of a baby. The neonatal intensive care unit (NICU) is a place of remarkable healing and recovery, and most babies do not die there. But, sometimes, despite everything, a baby will not live. We are so sorry if this has happened to you and your family. We are honored and grateful to Adrienne for sharing her memories in the following chapter. Even though your experience will be yours alone, we hope that her insight and advice will support you as you learn what to expect as your own story unfolds.

> A nurse sat in the room with us and it was very peaceful and quiet. Clara breathed for a while and then her breaths became inconsistent. Slowly, she went away. The very last thing I remember about her was a tiny tear that slid down her face and then she was gone.
>
> *Adrienne, mother of **Clara***

CHAPTER 11

The Loss of Your Baby

> "Remembering the day Clara was born is something I don't do very much anymore. We had an unplanned home birth after a very fast labor, and for some reason, she never breathed. She made it to the NICU, but the next day the doctors explained that she was not going to live. When I think of Clara, I do it with great care and affection. I've come to accept her short life and have stopped questioning why.
>
> *Adrienne, mother of* **Clara**"

There are few experiences in life as difficult as the heartbreaking death of a baby. As parents, you must face the loss of your baby and your dreams. You might also have to manage the practical details of the situation while continuing to support others who rely on you. This experience will change who you are and how you live. As this experience unfolds, please remember that *you* are your baby's parent. Although the opportunities to parent your baby may have been limited or very different from what you hoped, you will participate in the important decisions that affect you and your baby. Everything you do will help create the memory you will have for the rest of your life.

Difficult Choices for a Seriously Ill Baby

The birth of an extremely preterm baby or a baby with a significant health problem frequently raises many questions and requires parents to make difficult decisions. If the problem is known before your baby's birth, your doctors may have the chance to meet with you and have a detailed discussion about what to expect and what treatment options are available. Sometimes, a preterm birth happens quickly. Sometimes, a serious health problem isn't discovered until after birth or until a baby develops a life-threatening complication, and you will have an unexpected discussion with your baby's doctors. This can be very frightening. In either case, parents may have to make difficult choices about their baby's care.

Often, the outcome (*prognosis*) is not as certain, and the NICU team will work with you to make the best decisions for your baby's care. A baby may have problems that would require prolonged and uncomfortable treatment but still have only a small chance of survival. If the baby does survive, there may be serious problems that require lifelong care and limit the child's ability to enjoy everyday activities. In this case, you will work with the health care team to make very difficult decisions. The doctors, nurses, and other health care team members will explain your baby's problems and the potentially available treatments, and they will give you their best estimates of the treatment risks and possible outcomes. Some families put the highest value on any chance of their baby's survival, even if it means their baby could endure a long hospitalization and multiple procedures, and possibly survive with serious disabilities. Other families choose to spend a short amount of time with their baby, without medical devices, and limit the possibility of pain and suffering. Working together, your NICU team will be there for you to discuss your thoughts, your questions, and your beliefs and decide what type of treatment is best for your baby.

> " Our voice was honored all the way through. After Clara was admitted to the NICU, I needed surgery, so I couldn't be with Clara the night she was born, but my husband and his sister were with her. The NICU allowed them to do what they needed to move through this experience. They allowed them to take pictures, stay with her, talk to her, have her baptized. They supported our process without inserting their own agenda. The NICU staff remained silently supportive. "
>
> *Adrienne, mother of **Clara***

Together, you may decide to continue intensive life-sustaining treatment, to continue certain treatments but not others, or to stop life-sustaining treatment and focus on providing comfort and pain relief to your baby. If you decide to put limits on which treatments you want, the doctor may ask you to help write a care plan so all of your baby's caregivers know your wishes and goals and what treatments are acceptable. A *do not attempt resuscitation* (DNAR or DNR) *order* may be part of that plan. A DNAR order indicates you do not want emergency measures, like chest compressions (cardiopulmonary resuscitation) or emergency medications (such as epinephrine), used if your baby's heart stops beating or your baby stops breathing.

The decision to stop life-sustaining treatment and allow a baby to die comfortably is not made by a single person or by the parents alone. Like you, the NICU team wants what is best for your baby, and your input is essential. It is important that you understand the available treatment options and the possible risks and benefits of each option, and that you carefully consider what you believe is best for your baby. In most cases, there is no single right answer. Even though the NICU team may have faced a similar situation before, each baby and family are unique. Two families faced with the same situation may make completely different choices. What is most important is that you feel the decisions were right for your baby.

Considering the Decision to Stop Life-sustaining Therapy

When the NICU team asks to talk with you about making treatment decisions that include the possibility of stopping life-sustaining treatment, you may not be ready. You may even be shocked or angry that they asked. When facing this situation, ask as many questions as you need to, and then ask again to make sure you understand the answers. Some questions do not have answers, but the team will try to explain everything they can. You will find some suggestions to help you with this conversation on page 324.

Parents often feel a sense of relief after they reach agreement about such a difficult decision. At times, you will likely second-guess your decision and have some doubts, but these are normal feelings that will take time, and sometimes professional help, to resolve. This will certainly be one of the most difficult experiences you will ever go through, but you will not regret taking part in the decision-making process. If you and the NICU team determine that intensive medical treatment is prolonging suffering without any benefit, the focus of care for your baby will be directed toward providing comfort. Allowing your baby to have a peaceful and comfortable death is a choice that you make as loving parents who only want the best for your baby.

When Parents Have to Make Difficult Decisions

- Avoid getting critical information about your baby over the phone.

- Write down your questions as you think of them so you don't forget to ask later.

- Let the NICU team know who you would like to be with you during difficult conversations. Is there someone in your family or a support person you want to be with you? Are there topics that you don't want discussed in front of family members?

- If your baby's condition has a name, ask your doctor to write it down for you. You can ask what caused the problem. Sometimes, it is not any one specific condition that has led to your baby's critical situation but a series of complications resulting from the original problem.

- Ask your doctor to explain the condition. What are the treatment choices? Can the outcome of each choice be predicted?

- If necessary, remind the NICU team to use words that you understand and to talk at a pace that allows you to consider the information and ask questions.

- Tell your NICU team if there are cultural or religious factors that influence your decision-making process or practices that are important to you in this situation.

- Take your time. Let your doctor know when you are overwhelmed with information and need a break. This also gives you time to think of questions and write them down.

- Repeat the information in your own words to make sure you understand what you have been told.

- If English is not your preferred language, ask for a medical translator. Do not use a family member, a friend, or a child to translate.

- In some cases, your doctor may be able to connect you to a family who has faced a similar decision and can provide some additional perspective for your decision-making.

Organ Donation

Organ donation may be a way of having something good come out of this terrible experience. Although it will not bring your baby back to you, it may allow someone else's baby to live. Neonatal organ donation is a very personal and emotional decision.

If your baby is dying and you would like to consider organ donation, talk to your baby's doctor. Babies who die in the NICU may not be eligible to become organ donors because of their size or the time between stopping life support and the baby's death. Your doctor will contact the agency responsible for organ donation in your area and find out if your baby meets the criteria. If your baby does meet the criteria, a counselor from the organ donation agency will talk with you about the possibility.

Preparing to Say Farewell

You may feel very alone during this time. We hope that you are surrounded by supportive family and friends who can help you through this difficult experience.

Reuniting the Birthing Parent and Baby

If your baby was transported to a NICU in another hospital, both parents may not be in the NICU when difficult decisions are made or when your baby is near death. Ask your NICU team what can be done to bring the birthing parent and baby together. If you are the birthing parent and are in a medically stable condition, an early hospital discharge may be arranged. If your insurance allows, a birthing parent may also be medically transferred to the hospital where the baby is receiving care.

Naming Your Baby

If you have not yet done so, consider giving your baby a name. Naming your baby will help you and others recognize that your baby has a place in the story of your life. Naming your baby also establishes a memory that you will be able to reflect on later. Referring to a baby by name, even after death, gives dignity to that life.

Family Participation

The NICU staff will encourage family members, including older siblings, to be together as a family when a baby dies. Spending time with your baby gives family members the opportunity to know your baby and create their own memories. This is also the opportunity to incorporate your family traditions or spiritual customs into your baby's life. With your permission, religious clergy are always welcome in the NICU. The hospital's chaplaincy service can accommodate many different traditions and may be able to help if you prefer clergy of a specific denomination.

Events may occur quickly. Birth, death, and funeral may take place within a span of a few days. Experiencing this tragedy as a family will help everyone get through it. In addition, when the family talks about the baby in the future, all family members who participated will be able to share their memories and support.

Bringing Your Baby Home to Die

Not all babies with incurable conditions require a lot of technological support. You may consider taking your baby home to die. If you are considering this, talk with your NICU team about what you would like to do and learn about the rules and regulations in your state that affect your options. If it is possible to take your baby home to die and you decide to do so, the NICU team will help you develop a home care plan, teach you what to expect as your baby's condition changes, and provide a contact person who will always be available to answer questions and give support.

Near the Time of Death

When your baby is dying, the main priority is the baby's comfort and companionship. If you are in the NICU, the staff will arrange for you to hold your baby, preferably in a private, quiet area. Many of the tubes, wires, and medical equipment may have been removed so you can hold your baby closely without interference. This may be the first time you are able to hold and care for your baby without wires and tubes getting in the way.

The NICU staff will tell you what you can expect to see, hear, and feel as you hold your baby. You may ask someone from the staff to stay with you or just to be available if you call. This is important parenting time, so do not feel pressured or hurried. Someone from the NICU team will listen to your baby's heartbeat every so often with a stethoscope to determine the time of death. Sometimes, babies die very quickly after life support equipment is removed, but other times, babies have a slow heartbeat and take occasional breaths for a long time. While comforting your baby, let someone know if you need to take a break.

> " The role the nurses, doctors, and social workers played at the hospital was significant. Our ability to move through this experience in the most positive way was made possible by their nurturing and guidance. They took the best care of Clara and all of us. They guided our decisions with their knowledge and experience and captured the important memories for us to hold onto. My entire family is forever thankful and we still remember everyone at the hospital with the fondest of memories. "

Adrienne, mother of **Clara**

> ❝ We still have the memory book with her hair and prints and measurements. It brings such joy to my heart knowing that the nurses took the time to record her short life and treat her so well. ❞
>
> *Adrienne, mother of **Clara***

Preparing Memories

The NICU staff will help you prepare memories of your baby. Many parents want to take photographs and hold their baby for a family portrait. Some NICUs have an arrangement with a hospital-based or professional photographer specially trained to take these photos. Tell the NICU staff if you have special clothes or a blanket that you want your baby wrapped in for the photos. Some families think they don't want photos or aren't ready to take them home right away. You can still ask the staff to take photographs and save them at the hospital until you are ready to receive them some time after your baby's death.

Many NICUs will help you prepare a memory box including such things as the blankets and clothing you brought in, footprints, the hospital ID bracelet, a tape measure, the baby's crib card, and even a lock of hair. You may find all of this comforting, but if you do not, consider keeping these items in case you decide you want them later on.

After Death

After your baby has died, you still have all the time you need to say good-bye. When you are ready, your baby's nurse will undress your baby and prepare your baby to be carried to the hospital morgue. It is common for nurses to bathe the baby before leaving the NICU, and you are welcome to help or give the bath yourself. Doing something like this for your baby may help you say good-bye, but don't feel you must if it makes you uncomfortable. After the bath, you may want to rock and hold your baby again. After you have said good-bye, your baby will receive special identification tags and be carried to the morgue.

> Depending on your situation, this might be the only time you will ever spend with your baby. Take the time to hold, look at, and talk to your baby. Take pictures. You don't want to rush through this because when you look back, these memories will be all you have. I can't stress this enough, as it is my big and only regret. I was too quick to end the moment because it was so painful. When I look back and when we celebrate Clara's birthdays, the only wish I have is that I would have sat with her longer, talked to her, and been with her longer. In fact, when asked if there was one wish I could have come true, that wish is to go back and sit in that room with her one more time.

Adrienne, mother of **Clara**

Taking the Next Steps

After your baby has died, you will be asked to consider some additional choices. If you are having difficulty, call on those who have helped and supported you up until now—your nurses, doctors, family, friends, social workers, and clergy.

Considering an Autopsy

After your baby dies, a member of the NICU team will ask you to consider an autopsy. An autopsy, or postmortem examination, can provide valuable information that helps you understand why your baby died and identify any additional problems that weren't known before death. Sometimes, the results will provide information that might be useful when thinking about future pregnancies for you or your relatives.

If your baby died in a small hospital, your doctor may ask to have the autopsy performed at a neighboring medical center or children's hospital. The early results may be known in a few days, but the detailed results can take 6 or more weeks. Usually, the doctor who cared for your baby will meet with you, explain the results, and, if you wish, give you a copy of the report.

Funeral Arrangements and Transport

A funeral will let you, your family, and your close friends say good-bye to your baby in a public way as a celebration of your baby's short life. It also allows public recognition that this was a person who lived and had a profound influence on other people's lives.

After your baby's death, you will be asked to identify a funeral home whose staff will help to make all of the other arrangements. Your NICU social worker, family support representative, or grief counselor may be able to provide a list of area funeral homes and other available resources. If you are not sure what kind of ceremony is right for you and your baby, talk with the professionals at the funeral home. If your baby dies far from where you live, the funeral home can help you arrange transport, if needed.

Talking With Friends

As painful as it may be, you'll need to tell your close friends what happened. If your baby's life was very short, friends may not even know that your baby was born. This may be your first chance to speak with them about your baby. Calling close friends helps mobilize support, validates your feelings of loss as they express their shock and grief, and helps you find a way to live with this loss. If you wish, ask family members or a few close friends to pass the news to other friends. This relieves you of endless phone calls.

Understanding Grief

It's important to recognize that no 2 people grieve the same way. Not everyone experiences all of the stages of the grief process, and people experiencing the same loss may not experience the stages at the same time or in the same way.

At this point in your life, it may seem that nothing will ever make you feel good again. No one can tell you exactly how to get through this experience, but you may find some of the following suggestions helpful. If you have previously experienced a loss or have survived crises, try to recall what helped you most in that situation. Was it spending time with a friend? Attending a group session? Also, try to maintain your usual daily habits, even if you are unable to sleep. A sense of routine may help you feel more normal and less "lost."

Differences in How Parents Grieve

Parents often grieve differently. One parent may feel as though they must continue to take care of their family's needs, physically and emotionally. The other parent may feel as though they are expected to be strong and unemotional in a crisis. They may appear distant and quiet as they try to suppress their emotions. In the past, the non-birthing parent was given less attention during the grieving process because of the erroneous belief that they do not experience the same loss as the birthing parent. Allowing both parents to grieve openly may help them resolve their grief.

Sometimes, one parent will return to work soon after the death of a baby. When they focus on their work, it may appear they are not grieving or have moved beyond their grief. Neither may be true. The difference in behaviors may be that they are not alone all day focusing on their grief. When they come home, they may need to set aside their own grief to provide support to a grieving partner or child.

Lack of communication between parents is one of the reasons for the high divorce rate among couples who have lost a baby. The loss of a baby may be the first major crisis a couple faces together. It can be frightening to see your partner lose control, and it may be difficult to deal with a crisis if both of you are lost, overwhelmed, and unable to support each other. The stress is great, and the potential for misunderstanding each other is high. It's helpful if couples talk over small misunderstandings before they become insurmountable problems.

Coping Strategies

During this time, you may find relief by expressing yourself artistically. This serves 2 purposes. First, it can help you sort through your emotions day by day. Second, when everything is over and for many years to come, your work will provide you with remembrances of a bittersweet time. Some creative coping strategies include writing (for example, letters to your baby, poetry, a journal, blogging), scrapbooking, drawing, painting, creating pottery, or sculpting. It is entirely up to you whether you share these outlets or keep them private.

Some parents find comfort by joining a parent support group. Sometimes, talking to others who have experienced the same or a similar event is very helpful. The NICU social worker can give you more information.

> After Clara's funeral, they allowed me to come back and meet all of the nurses and doctors who tended to Clara in the NICU. That was a very healing day for me. I wanted to meet and talk to the people who spent more time with her than I did. They shared little tidbits and cared enough to tell me everything they could remember about Clara and how she may have touched their lives. I took the time to thank them and tell them I knew they did everything short of being God to keep her alive. I felt there wasn't a single thing that could have been done differently and that was so comforting. I would hate to be grieving while thinking there was something more that could have been done—that would have been torture. Their support went above and beyond any expectation I could have had.

*Adrienne, mother of **Clara***

Loss of a Twin or Other Multiple

Multiple-gestation births can be a special event, but parents who lose one child from a set of twins or other multiple births face a unique situation. The loss of one child is not made up for by the survival of another. The child who is lost is always missed and always mourned, even if only privately.

Caring for the surviving twin may be a source of sadness and joy. Your emotions are on a roller-coaster ride as you celebrate the birth and life of a healthy baby and grieve for what has been lost. Because of the turmoil surrounding the death of one baby, parents may feel like they are ignoring the needs of the other. They may feel guilty that they can only provide the basic needs of their other baby, such as feeding and diapering, but cannot attend to their emotional needs.

With time, a balance can be found. With time, many parents learn to be happy for the surviving baby and deal with that baby's problems while grieving for the baby who has died. Each parent reacts to the death of a multiple differently. The only way to get through the experience is to talk about it and respect each other's feelings.

Helping Others Cope With Grief

Coping with your own feelings may seem like all you can do right now, but as you move through your grief, you may find yourself supporting those around you.

Grandparents

Your baby's grandparents will grieve in their own ways for their own reasons. Like parents, they grieve the loss of the future. Grandparents develop their own fantasies about their grandchild—what the baby will look like, what they will do together, what they hope the baby will become. When a grandchild dies or is severely disabled, grandparents also mourn the loss of that future.

In addition, grandparents hurt for you, their own children. They never stop being parents, and your pain compounds their grief. But don't overlook the support your parents offer. They may be separated enough from the situation to help you make plans and decisions.

Your Baby's Siblings

Sibling grief reactions vary, depending on the age of the sibling. Although younger children may not fully comprehend what has occurred, even the youngest child will sense the emotional turmoil surrounding the loss of the baby. Unlike adults, children do not grieve continuously. Much to your surprise, your children may be able to continue their daily routine and play and eat as usual. Then, when you least expect it, one of them may remember something about the baby and become very sad.

Some predictable grief reactions occur in children. They may feel guilty because they believe they caused their sibling's death or disability by wishful thinking. They may misbehave and regress in their behavior (for example, go back to thumb-sucking or bed-wetting). They may experience frightening thoughts that others are going to die. They may also be frightened by your strong emotions.

When explaining death to children, use real words and express the problems honestly. Children may need reassurance that the same thing will not happen to them. Avoid talking about death as going to sleep; that may result in sleeping problems. Be honest: "The baby was born too soon and she was too small"; "The baby was born very sick and she died"; and especially, "The baby's problems are nobody's fault."

Be as honest as possible with your children without going into too much detail. Answer questions concisely with as much explanation as you feel is appropriate. It's all right to admit that you don't have all the answers. Resources are available to assist you, but remember— you know your children best. Trust your instincts as you struggle with what to say.

Like adults, children are unique and may grieve in unique ways. An unconcerned attitude that continues without any change, however, may be a signal that your child is denying the situation or is unable to express their emotions. Your child may benefit from professional counseling in dealing with the feelings.

Friends

You may have friends who were—or are still—pregnant at this time. Seeing these friends can be especially challenging after your baby has died. Friends may respond to your loss in a number of ways. Some who are sad and scared for you may withdraw simply because they do not know what to do or say. Others may be more comfortable with your grief, stay close, and support you through this difficult time.

Many people have difficulty speaking to mourning parents and say nothing or the wrong thing. You will probably encounter many well-intentioned people with a knack for saying the wrong thing: "You're young; you can have others"; "This happened for the best"; and, "At least you still have one of the twins." You will probably also have dear, close friends who realize that saying "I'm sorry" or "We're thinking of you," or whose presence alone, is a great comfort to you.

Duration of Grief

Your life has now changed forever, but you will eventually find a new place of emotional peace where you feel comfortable and belong.

When to Get Help for Your Grief

Throughout the grief process, you may wonder if you are normal. You may wonder if you have been sad, angry, or feeling confused for too long. Most people are able to work through their grief with help from their partner, family members, friends, and coworkers. However, you may want to obtain help from a therapist, family counselor, social worker, or another professional if you feel you need it or if any of the following situations occur:

- You are afraid you may physically harm yourself or someone else; you have thoughts of suicide.
- You are participating in activities that may damage your health (for example, drugs, alcohol, overeating, not eating enough).
- The support of friends and family members is not enough.
- You experience more losses after the death of your baby.
- You think very poorly of yourself and feel out of control, depressed, or stressed out all the time.

People grieve at their own pace. The first year is usually one of experiencing all of the "firsts," living a full year of special dates (birthdays and holidays), and feeling the acute pain of your loss as these dates occur. Even though your baby's death may not affect how your family celebrates a particular event, you may feel your loss most at family gatherings.

The second year is usually spent looking toward the future, reorganizing your life without your baby in it. As time passes, your loss will feel less physically painful, and you'll learn to laugh again. Expect to experience occasional "blue" days, when some date or event causes you to reexperience your grief. Your grief may come and go over time, and small remembrances may trigger strong feelings of grief again. If you feel you are too sad for too long, consider speaking with your own doctor or a mental health professional.

One of the most challenging considerations for parents who have lost a child is how to answer the innocent question, "How many children do you have?" Your answer to this question may change over time, and you may have different replies in different circumstances. This is completely acceptable, and you will learn what is most comfortable for you.

> ❝ We have another child, a boy, who was born 16 months after Clara. I have always felt her spirit in him, like a little dancing angel who twinkles through at the most unexpected times. I am at peace. ❞
>
> *Adrienne, mother of* **Clara**

A Bittersweet Time

Few things in life are more difficult than making decisions for a critically ill or dying baby. Drawing on the love and support of family, friends, and the NICU health care team will help you make the choices that will ultimately be best for you and your child.

It may take time for your decisions to feel completely right. The choices facing you are complex and will awaken many new emotions. As time goes by, though, you'll be thankful you were empowered to make these choices for your baby and grateful you were able to control some aspects of this overwhelming time in your life.

Appendix

· · · · · ·

Where Are They Now?

We caught up with some of the families from the first edition of *Understanding the NICU.* See how they are doing now.

Sienna, 31 weeks, 4 days

Sienna is 13 years old and flourishing during her 7th grade year! She has found a love for basketball, volleyball, and track. It's no surprise to us that she is fast, considering how quickly she was born into this world!

She is a big sister to two little brothers and a little sister. She is such a great friend, and she loves her family fiercely.

Sienna is healthy and thriving. She warms everyone's heart with her big smile and genuine laugh. We credit her resiliency and ability to exceed our expectations in all areas of life to the excellent care she received in the NICU. She showed us at a young age that she is, and always will be, a NICU warrior.

Kaitlynn, mother of Sienna

Sienna.

Pascal, 41 weeks, 2 days

Pascal is 7 years old now and doing well. He no longer has any medical complications and is doing well in school. My PTSD, however, is long-lasting, and I worry that it has affected my ability to parent him.

I would find myself so consumed by worrying—is he going to fall off that slide? He's going to fall off that slide, and we'll have to go to the hospital. Who will I call to help? How will I get him into his car seat?—that I had nothing left for the realities of his toddlerhood and his intense 3s and 4s. Medications have helped me, but I still wonder if it affected our relationship.

I'm much more patient with his little brother, who was late preterm but had no NICU stay. I wish there had been more awareness in the NICU of the emotional impact on parents, and more resources available after we went home. It took me a year to get help for myself, and that was just completely unnecessary.

My advice to NICU parents would be to advocate not only for your baby, but for yourself. If you suffer from anxiety that doesn't go away or interferes with your daily life, or your ability to be the parent you want to be, tell someone and get help. The sooner you get help, the sooner you'll be on your way to recovery.

Alex, father of Pascal

August (Auggie), 24 weeks

August is almost 10 years old now and thriving as a happy, healthy, precocious little boy. He enjoys spending time with his friends, LOVES reading, telling jokes, riding his bike, walking his 2 Labrador Retrievers, swimming, fishing, watching science fiction movies, and going on

all kinds of adventures with us, his parents. All of his well-visit checkups over the past 5 years have been "unremarkable" in the sense that his start as a very premature baby is now irrelevant to anything needing discussion. He's been extremely healthy, all around, and for that we remain forever grateful.

Our time in the NICU is a distant memory, and the pain and anguish are very much gone. Still, though, this experience not only makes us grateful for his wonderful health status now, but also deeply compassionate toward those parents who are still going through this challenging and uncertain time and for those who continue to feel these intense emotions after their baby comes home.

Auggie.

The NICU experience is one of hope and resiliency. For us, the deep emotions and feelings of guilt and sadness have faded. Instead, we are left with a great appreciation for the field of neonatology, the clinicians and larger caregiving teams, and families' abilities to overcome such a challenging and traumatic start to life.

Robyn, mother of Auggie

 Lucy, 29 weeks

It is honestly hard to believe when we look at Lucy that she was once a tiny baby spending many long days and nights in the NICU. I remember her physical therapist in the NICU telling me

on one of those long days that although it sometimes feels like you will never leave the NICU, that it will one day be just a blip in your journey. And she was right. It feels as if we blinked, life shifted, and we now have a second grader! Lucy is 8 years old and is an amazing big sister to Elliott (who is 5 and followed in Lucy's footsteps as a preemie born at 35 weeks). Lucy is a voracious reader, naturally talented at riding a bike, and just starred in her first play! She is tall and smart and strong willed and makes friends wherever she goes. We talk regularly with Lucy about her NICU time and about what an incredible fighter she has always been and continues to be.

Lucy.

Lucy understands that her body has some limitations that other kids do not have, and she talks openly about it and doesn't shy away from advocating for herself. Eight is truly a magical age and we are so thankful for her journey and the person she has developed into over the years. There is also something very strange about getting to know your child when they arrive early. Many people may not realize the fierce personalities that NICU babies already have but I still will see glimpses of moments with Lucy in the NICU especially her sense of humor and determination. And still to this day, Lucy does things according to Lucy's timeline—just as she did back in the NICU.

Kate and Matt, parents of Lucy

 ## Niklas, Gabbie, and Lukas, 28 weeks, 4 days

Our trio is great, really great. They are sophomores in high school where they are straight A students. Lukas has been swimming on the local swim team since first grade. Niklas is a short

 distance runner (missed going to the State meet by a hair this year), and Gabbie trains horses. All 3 of them play 2 different musical instruments. They are 16 years old now and taller than me. We are so lucky!

Jason and Greta, parents of Niklas, Gabbie, & Lukas

Niklas, Gabbie, & Lukas.

 ## Allison and Reece, 33 weeks

Allison and Reece have no lingering effects of their early birth. They have academically hit all their milestones and are getting ready to start middle school in the fall. Reece is an avid lacrosse player who enjoys learning new magic card tricks, riding his bike, and meeting up

 with friends. Allison is a skilled archer who went to the Nationals tournament last year and enjoys taking gymnastics classes and being active with her Girl Scout troop. She is excited to start cheerleading later this year. We are forever thankful to the NICU doctors and nurses who helped our twins through the scary times and gave them the best possible start to their lives.

Allison & Reece.

Gudrun, mother of Allison & Reece

Kellan, 32 weeks

It's hard to believe that it has been 10 years since our first child was born at just 32 weeks' gestation! Kellan continues to thrive. He is in fifth grade, pitching and playing first base on a travel

 baseball team, golfing at every opportunity, teasing his younger sister constantly, and really gaining a sense of independence. We are so proud of all he has overcome and can't wait to see the amazing things he has yet to accomplish. Forever grateful for our NICU family for making it all possible.

Marnie, mother of Kellan

Kellan.

 Frankie, 29 weeks

Frankie, now approaching her tenth trip around the sun, is active, healthy, and thriving. She loves a challenging adventure whether that is getting lost in a wonderful book about spirit animals, building robots, or hiking to the top of Mt. Ellinor. She plays soccer, rides her bike, swims, snow

 skis, and has a real appreciation for an active lifestyle. She adores her pets and is genuinely kind to everyone. It was no shock to watch our super preemie's fascination and success in math and science. She absolutely loves learning and loves school.

Ten years ago, we weren't exactly sure if she was going to survive. As we watched her grow and develop that first year, we wondered what challenges she would face. She came into the world early. She was shockingly small. She

Frankie. had challenges with eating, and her issues with silent reflux were painful and heartbreaking. We stayed the course. We focused on meeting her needs. She made positive progress in growth. She finally enjoyed eating. And every single day she made strides and gains in cognitive development, fine and gross motor skills, speech and language, and social and emotional development. Frankie the Super Preemie is Frankie.

We no longer worry about the preemie stuff. We are forever grateful for science, and the people who cared for and protected our greatest gift, a healthy child. She is so fortunate to have 2 all-in parents, an incredible pediatrician, smart and caring teachers, motivating coaches, fun friends, and a loving family that has and continues to contribute to her success and development. I have whispered and repeated our mantra since the day she was born: "No Barriers," and she has certainly proven that.

Lisa, mother of Frankie

Jack, 29 weeks, and Henry, 31 weeks

Jack and Henry are both doing amazing! Jack is 13 and in the seventh grade where he excels academically. He enjoys playing Xbox with friends, skiing and basketball but has a real passion for cooking. He enjoys learning about new cuisines and has taken several cooking classes. Jack hopes to be on the culinary team in high school and go to Columbia University and live in New York City. He knows it's awhile away but he likes to dream big!

Jack. Henry.

Henry is 11 and enjoying fifth grade! He is still our "active" child who loves to run and play sports. Like his brother Jack, he enjoys skiing and hopes to be doing black diamonds this winter. He plays flag football and basketball, but his favorite sport is soccer. He has played since he was 3 and has been on the same team the last few years. He also has passion for helping others and recently held a fundraiser to raise money for kids in Ukraine.

Our time in the NICU feels like ages ago and I am still amazed at how well the kids have done considering their rough starts in life. We will forever be grateful to all the health care providers who were involved in their care! NICU kids are truly special!

Kristina, mother of Jack & Henry

Holland and Eden, 24 weeks, 3 days

It's hard to believe that Holland and Eden have celebrated their 18th birthdays and are in their senior year of high school! Along with the rest of the world, we faced a lot of challenges these past few years with the pandemic, virtual schooling, isolation, and health-related worries. We

are very thankful that we were able to make it through the worst of it relatively unscathed. The girls transferred to a new high school this year that ended up being exactly what they needed with a smaller setting, more individualized attention, and a really wonderful and supportive group of friends, teachers, and staff. Both girls are growing, learning, and making progress at their own pace and in their own unique ways.

Our family. Back row: Holland, Dad, and Mom. Front row: Pidge the dog, Violet, and Eden.

Holland volunteers at our local humane society and enjoys spending time socializing and cuddling with cats during her weekly sessions. She also started therapeutic riding and loves learning to ride, groom, and connect with the horses at the barn. She continues to love Pokémon and all things Marvel. She spends her free time playing video games, hanging out with our dog Pidge, watching her favorite YouTube and Twitch streamers, watching anime, and chatting with her friends on Discord.

Eden does well in school, doing dual enrollment at a local community college and maintaining a 4.0 grade point average. She has been very involved as the secretary of the high school anime club and helped pull together a successful anime convention. She also enjoys spending time with her boyfriend, horseback riding, connecting with friends in virtual reality, digital art, and exploring different genres of music. Her love of Japanese culture endures, and we are planning a trip to Tokyo during their senior year.

Our "take home baby" and littlest sister Violet is in fifth grade and following in her big sisters' footsteps when it comes to her love of video games, movies, and books! Violet is also active with dance, Girl Scouts, and watching make-up tutorials online.

All 3 girls share a deep connection with and love for their family, and we feel so lucky to have these wonderful people in our lives! Even after 18 years, those early NICU days and all that they went through to survive are never far from our minds, and we are eternally grateful to the staff who helped care for them (and us) during that time.

Billie, mother of Holland & Eden

Conversion of Pounds, Ounces, and Grams

Find the baby's weight in pounds down the left side of the table. Find the ounces across the top of the table. The intersection of the 2 measurements equals the equivalent weight in grams. For example, 3 pounds 8 ounces equals 1,588 g. To convert grams to pounds and ounces, find the baby's weight in grams. Look to the far left line for the pounds and to the top of the gram column for the ounces. For example, 1,134 g equals 2 pounds 8 ounces.

CONVERSION OF POUNDS AND OUNCES TO GRAMS

Pounds \ Ounces	0	1	2	3	4	5	6	7	8	9	10	11	12	13	14	15
0	—	28	57	85	113	142	170	198	227	255	283	312	340	369	397	425
1	454	482	510	539	567	595	624	652	680	709	737	765	794	822	850	879
2	907	936	964	992	1,021	1,049	1,077	1,106	1,134	1,162	1,191	1,219	1,247	1,276	1,304	1,332
3	1,361	1,389	1,417	1,446	1,474	1,502	1,531	1,559	1,588	1,616	1,644	1,673	1,701	1,729	1,758	1,786
4	1,814	1,843	1,871	1,899	1,928	1,956	1,984	2,013	2,041	2,070	2,098	2,126	2,155	2,183	2,211	2,240
5	2,268	2,296	2,325	2,353	2,381	2,410	2,438	2,466	2,495	2,523	2,551	2,580	2,608	2,637	2,665	2,693
6	2,722	2,750	2,778	2,807	2,835	2,863	2,892	2,920	2,948	2,977	3,005	3,033	3,062	3,090	3,118	3,147
7	3,175	3,203	3,232	3,260	3,289	3,317	3,345	3,374	3,402	3,430	3,459	3,487	3,515	3,544	3,572	3,600
8	3,629	3,657	3,685	3,714	3,742	3,770	3,799	3,827	3,856	3,884	3,912	3,941	3,969	3,997	4,026	4,054
9	4,082	4,111	4,139	4,167	4,196	4,224	4,252	4,281	4,309	4,337	4,366	4,394	4,423	4,451	4,479	4,508
10	4,536	4,564	4,593	4,621	4,649	4,678	4,706	4,734	4,763	4,791	4,819	4,848	4,876	4,904	4,933	4,961
11	4,990	5,018	5,046	5,075	5103	5,131	5,160	5,188	5,216	5,245	5,273	5,301	5,330	5,358	5,386	5,415
12	5,443	5,471	5,500	5,528	5,557	5,585	5,613	5,642	5,670	5,698	5,727	5,755	5,783	5,812	5,840	5,868

CONVERSION OF CENTIMETERS TO INCHES					
Centimeters	**Inches**	**Centimeters**	**Inches**	**Centimeters**	**Inches**
25.4	10	43.2	17	61.0	24
26.7	10½	44.4	17½	62.2	24½
27.9	11	45.7	18	63.5	25
29.2	11½	47.0	18½	64.8	25½
30.5	12	48.3	19	66.1	26
31.8	12½	49.5	19½	67.4	26½
33.0	13	50.8	20	68.7	27
34.3	13½	52.1	20½	69.9	27½
35.6	14	53.3	21	71.2	28
36.8	14½	54.6	21½	72.5	28½
38.1	15	55.9	22	73.8	29
39.4	15½	57.2	22½	75.1	29½
40.6	16	58.4	23	76.4	30
41.9	16½	59.7	23½	77.6	30½

CONVERSION OF TEMPERATURE (FAHRENHEIT AND CELSIUS)	
Under most circumstances, a normal target range for a newborn's temperature is about 36.5°C to 37.5°C (97.7°F–99.5°F).	
Fahrenheit	**Celsius**
96.1	35.6
96.4	35.8
96.8	36.0
97.7	36.5
98.6	37.0
99.5	37.5
100.4	38.0
101.3	38.5
102.2	39.0
103.1	39.5
104.0	40.0
104.9	40.5
105.8	41.0
106.7	41.5
107.6	42.0

Expanded Apgar Score   Gestational Age _____ weeks

Sign	0	1	2	1 min	5 min	10 min	15 min	20 min
Color	Blue or pale	Acrocyanotic	Completely pink					
Heart rate	Absent	<100 bpm	>100 bpm					
Reflex irritability	No response	Grimace	Cry or active withdrawal					
Muscle tone	Limp	Some flexion	Active motion					
Respiration	Absent	Weak cry, hypoventilation	Good, crying					
			TOTAL					

Comments	Resuscitation					
	Min	1	5	10	15	20
	Oxygen					
	PPV/NCPAP					
	ETT					
	Chest compressions					
	Epinephrine					

From American Academy of Pediatrics Committee on Fetus and Newborn, American College of Obstetricians and Gynecologists Committee on Obstetric Practice. The Apgar score. Pediatrics. 2015; 136 (4): 819-822. Reprinted with permission from: The Apgar score. Committee Opinion No. 644. American College of Obstetricians and Gynecologists. *Obstet Gynecol*. 2015;126e:e52–e55.

Index

● ● ● ●